A Practical Guide to Medicines Administration

It is important that medicines ⸺⸺⸺⸺⸺⸺⸺⸺⸺, in order to provide correct drug doses, yet not all healthcare professionals are experts in the area. This accessible book provides a definitive guide to best practice in administering medicinal formulations.

Acting as a quick reference handbook for administration techniques in both the simulated and real practice environment, the book enables readers to advise patients on the correct use of their formulation. It covers the following formulation types:

- oral
- topical
- ocular
- aural
- nasal
- inhaled
- transdermal patches
- vaginal
- rectal.

A Practical Guide to Medicines Administration is a key resource for both student and practising pharmacists who counsel and advise patients on the use of their medicines. It will also be a useful reference for nurses, nursing associates, assistant practitioners and healthcare assistants.

Karen Anne Gunnell is a Teaching Fellow in Pharmacy Practice at Keele University, UK.

Rebecca Hayley Venables is a Lecturer in Clinical Pharmacy at Keele University, UK.

A Practical Guide to Medicines Administration

Karen Anne Gunnell
and
Rebecca Hayley Venables

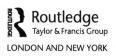

Routledge
Taylor & Francis Group

LONDON AND NEW YORK

First published 2019
by Routledge
2 Park Square, Milton Park, Abingdon, Oxon OX14 4RN

and by Routledge
711 Third Avenue, New York, NY 10017

Routledge is an imprint of the Taylor & Francis Group, an informa business

British Library Cataloguing-in-Publication Data
A catalogue record for this book is available from the British Library

Library of Congress Cataloging-in-Publication Data
Names: Gunnell, Karen Anne, author. | Venables, Rebecca Hayley, author.
Title: A practical guide to medicines administration / Karen Anne Gunnell
    and Rebecca Hayley Venables.
Description: Abingdon, Oxon ; New York, NY : Routledge, 2018. |
    Includes bibliographical references and index.
Identifiers: LCCN 2018009964| ISBN 9781138301160 (hardback) |
    ISBN 9781138301177 (paperback) | ISBN 9780203732717 (ebook)
Subjects: | MESH: Drug Administration Routes | Dosage Forms |
    Pharmaceutical Preparations—administration & dosage
Classification: LCC RM147 | NLM WB 340 | DDC 615/.6—dc23
LC record available at https://lccn.loc.gov/2018009964

ISBN: 978-1-138-30116-0 (hbk)
ISBN: 978-1-138-30117-7 (pbk)
ISBN: 978-0-203-73271-7 (ebk)

Typeset in Stempel Garamond
by Swales & Willis Ltd, Exeter, Devon, UK

Contents

The authors
We would like to thank Jaspreet Bharaj, for her illustrative creations.

Karen Anne Gunnell
I would like to thank my partner Steve and my family for your
ongoing support in everything I do. This book is for you.

Rebecca Hayley Venables
I am indebted to my dear family and friends for their patience,
ongoing support and encouragement.

Author biographies

Karen Anne Gunnell

Academic and community pharmacist Karen Anne Gunnell graduated with a Master of Pharmacy from Aston University, Birmingham, UK, in 2003. After completing her pre-registration training with Rowlands Pharmacy, she went on to manage one of their stores in Herefordshire. In 2007, she moved to Boots UK, where she went on to have a number of roles, including Divisional Care Homes Pharmacist, eLearning designer and teacher practitioner based at Keele University. In 2015, Karen moved to her present role at Keele University, to teach on the undergraduate MPharm and postgraduate diploma in Community Pharmacy courses. Karen has a postgraduate diploma in Clinical Pharmacy with Medicines Management from De Montford University and a postgraduate certificate in Teaching and Learning in Higher Education from Keele University. She is currently chair of the Education and Development Committee of UKCPA and is secretary of RPS Shropshire and Staffordshire Steering Committee. Karen is a Fellow of the Higher Education Academy.

Rebecca Hayley Venables

Dr Rebecca Hayley Venables graduated with a Master of Pharmacy from Aston University, Birmingham, UK in 2007. After completing her pre-registration training with Boots Pharmacy, she undertook a PhD in paediatric medicines adherence and gained her doctorate from the University of Birmingham, UK, in 2013. Whilst studying for her PhD, Rebecca continued to practise as a community pharmacist. In 2013, Rebecca joined Keele University as a Lecturer in Clinical Pharmacy and continues to practise as both an academic and community pharmacist today. She has a postgraduate certificate in Teaching and Learning in Higher Education from Keele University and has published research within the field of medicines adherence in paediatric patients. Rebecca is a Fellow of the Higher Education Academy. She is currently undertaking a master's degree in Teaching and Learning in Higher Education.

Introduction

A recent study has shown that only 7% of healthcare professionals could demonstrate the correct usage of an MDI (metered-dose inhaler).[1] Pharmacists are in the best place within the patient-facing environment to provide information on optimal formulation administration techniques. It is vital to ensure that such techniques are performed accurately in order to provide correct drug doses, and thus to minimise sub-therapeutic responses and also to promote safety (through reduction of overdose and also promoting points of good practice – one example would be to wash hands before using sterile eye drops, in order to avoid infection).

This book was originally designed to help MPharm undergraduate students completing advice-giving stations in their competency-based assessments, as it was identified that the requisite information was unavailable within one resource. This book is an invaluable resource for pre-registration and qualified pharmacists, trainee and qualified nurses, medical students, doctors, healthcare assistants and pharmacy support staff when counselling and advising patients on the use of their medicines. It is also a useful resource for care home employees when administering medicines.

Each chapter contains an introduction to the formulation, with information about the formulation type and pertinent key practice points. A list of administration instructions is provided. This details the key steps and best practice points involved with administering each formulation in order to provide safe and effective medicines use.

This book is designed to be a pocket companion of administration techniques for using common medicinal formulations. It is not designed to be read cover to cover, but instead to pick up and to put down, as required, for quick reference. This book is not designed to go into significant scientific detail, and there are other resources available that expand upon the concepts described.

In this book the authors have used the patient as the main recipient of advice. However, it may be necessary to advise carers, parents or guardians to ensure that the patient receives effective and safe treatment. The authors have written this book with the adult patient in mind (unless otherwise stated within the chapters), as different techniques may be recommended for children under 16 years of age. This book is not intended to replace manufacturers' patient information leaflets and product-specific information. However, it forms a basis for advice-giving consultations and medicine administration techniques.

Reference

1 Baverstock M, Woodhall N, Maarman V. Do healthcare professionals have sufficient knowledge of inhaler techniques in order to educate their patients effectively in their use? *Thorax* 2010;65:A117. doi: 10.1136/thx.2010.150979.45

Oral formulations

In the UK, the oral route of drug administration is used commonly. Oral formulations include: tablets (including chewable, soluble and oro-dispersible tablets), capsules, liquids (including syrups and suspensions), sublingual tablets and sprays, buccal tablets and liquids, lozenges and gums, and oral granules and powders.

Tablets and capsules

This chapter outlines a practical method for swallowing tablets and capsules. However, there are a number of techniques that may be employed if this method is unsuccessful. These may include:

- adding some soft food to your mouth and swallowing the food and tablet/capsule together
- drinking water through a straw when swallowing the tablet/capsule
- inserting the tablet/capsule into a cube of bread or other soft food item, e.g. yoghurt, and swallowing together.[1]

Some medication interacts or is incompatible with certain foodstuffs; therefore it is important to check with the summary of product characteristics (SPC) or the patient information leaflet to ensure safe and effective administration.

Some tablets have coatings that influence their release characteristics, e.g. film, sugar, enteric or modified release. These may have been designed to release the drug in the small intestine or to bypass drug release in the stomach. Coatings may also be used to protect the stomach from the drug, e.g. NSAIDs, or protect the drug from the acidic environment in the stomach, e.g. sulfasalazine. Some may also have been designed to release drug gradually over a prolonged period of time, e.g. diltiazem modified release tablets.

Tablets are available in chewable, oro-dispersible (allowed to dissolve on the tongue) and soluble versions. Although water is not needed to take oro-dispersible tablets, a lack of saliva may affect the rate of disintegration and dissolution.[2]

Oro-dispersible tablets are usually delicate and should be handled carefully, to avoid damaging the tablet prior to administration. They often come in packaging that requires additional mechanical strength to protect them and for the patient to peel back the film rather than 'popping' the tablet out.

Soluble tablets often have a high sodium content, which may be unsuitable for certain groups of patient, e.g. those with uncontrolled hypertension and renal disease.[3,4]

The benefits of tablets and capsules are that they are convenient and discreet; therefore they are favoured by many patients in the UK. Tablets can be designed to release drugs slowly and they are generally classed as relatively stable formulations, with regards to microbiology and their physical and chemical characteristics. They are relatively cheap to manufacture and have a long shelf-life.

A disadvantage of tablets is that they can be challenging for patient groups who have dysphagia or difficulties with swallowing. Taste masking can be difficult for certain drugs. Capsules may contain gelatine, derived from animals, which may be unacceptable to certain patient groups, e.g. vegetarians, vegans, some religious denominations.

Aids are available to crush or halve tablet formulations where necessary. This may be useful to ease administration, e.g. in patients with dysphagia, or to provide a dose that is not available commercially. Consideration should be made to formulations with coatings and special release mechanisms, as they may be less suitable for crushing and halving. In such circumstances, it is advisable to seek guidance from the relevant patient information leaflet.

Oral liquids

Oral liquids are particularly useful for administering drugs to some patient groups, e.g. the young and elderly, who have difficulties swallowing solid oral dosage forms. There are many different types of oral liquids, including: syrups, suspensions, solutions, drops, emulsions, mixtures, linctuses and elixirs. There are difficulties with oral liquids, such as increased formulation costs, manufacturing and distribution challenge. They often have short shelf-lives compared to solid oral dosage forms, and require further microbiological considerations. However, liquids do allow dosage flexibility and taste masking can be utilised.

When oral liquids are packaged in multi-dose containers, they may have different expiry dates once they have been opened. It is therefore recommended to refer to the specific manufacturer's instructions for this information. It is good practice to mark the container with the date of opening when dispensing or administering from a multi-dose container, as this will allow expiry dates to be observed.

Oral liquids, with the exception of homogenous solutions, should be shaken well before use. This will ensure uniformity of the product, and thus delivery of an accurate dose.

When liquids are poured into glass containers, they curve at the edges and down at the centre. To measure the accurate volume of a liquid, you should observe the level at which the meniscus (bottom of the curvature) sits. This should be measured at eye-line.

When pouring liquids to measure doses, it is good practice for the patient to place their hand over the label of the liquid. This helps to minimise liquid spillage, and therefore damage to the pharmacy label.

The conventional methods of administering oral liquids are via medicine spoon, oral syringe and measuring cup.

The 5mL spoon is the most commonly available medicine spoon. However, some medicine spoons are graduated and marked with doses other than the standard 5mL volume measurement. Patients should be advised to familiarise themselves with the graduations on medicine spoons to ensure optimal and safe dosing. In addition, some spoons have a smaller end with a capacity to measure a volume of 2.5mL. This may be used or, alternatively, an oral syringe may be preferred. When measuring liquid doses using a medicine spoon, it is recommended to measure a level spoonful to avoid spillages and promote accurate dosing. Patients should only use the provided medicine spoons when prescribed a dose of 'a spoonful'. This is because research has shown that household teaspoons can vary in volume capacity from 2.5mL to 7.3mL.[5]

Oral syringes are available in different sizes with different dosing graduations. The most common oral syringes available are 1mL and 5mL. The patient should be advised to carefully observe the dosing graduations and units on the oral syringe that they are using. Dosing graduations can differ and manufacturers may also provide specific syringes with different dosing units (e.g. mg instead of mL), which may be used for ease of administration. When being washed and reused, the graduation marks on oral syringes may begin to fade. It is important that syringes are discarded and replaced when this occurs, to avoid inaccurate dosing and to optimise patient safety.

Measuring cups provide a convenient method for measuring some volumes greater than 5mL. The graduations provided on measuring cups can vary widely according to manufacturer, and may be based on commonly required doses of specific products. The patient should always check that the graduations meet their dosing needs. If not, an alternative device should be used.

Medicine spoons, oral syringes and measuring cups can be washed using warm soapy water and rinsed with potable water, unless the manufacturer's instructions state otherwise. When cleaning an oral syringe, it is advised that the patient pulls the plunger of the syringe out to draw up, then pushes it back in to expel the warm soapy water. This method should then be repeated with potable water.

The majority of liquids are packaged in multi-dose containers. However, there are some products available in unit-dose packaging, such as sachets containing liquids. The instructions for administering these are the same as those for administering liquids from multi-dose containers, with the exception that the dose does not need to be measured prior to administration.

Buccal formulations

Buccal administration allows the drug to pass directly into the bloodstream via the oral mucosa in the buccal cavity, avoiding first-pass metabolism. This can improve the bioavailability of some drugs and allows for a faster onset of action.

In this chapter, the administration of buccal tablets and liquids is discussed. Buccal tablets are convenient for both local and systemic administration of drugs. They can take time to dissolve in the mouth, but once this is complete they provide a rapid onset of action. Occasionally, local irritation can occur. It is advisable, therefore, to recommend that the patient moves the position of the buccal tablet on the gum.[6]

Midazolam is one example of a drug administered via a buccal liquid. It is predominantly used for status epilepticus. It is currently available in multi-dose bottles and unit-dose pre-filled syringes (the administration techniques for both are discussed in this chapter). When stored in the multi-dose bottles, midazolam should be a clear liquid without crystals. If crystals are visible in the product, the product should be discarded appropriately.[7] Note that not all formulations of midazolam currently have a product licence.

Sublingual formulations

Drugs administered via the sublingual route pass through the oral mucosa under the tongue. This permits a fast onset of action as first-pass metabolism is avoided. The sublingual method utilises tablets and sprays, both of which are discussed within this chapter.

Nitrates are often administered via the sublingual route for the treatment of angina. Some nitrate sprays contain alcohol and should therefore not be used near a naked flame.

Gum and lozenges

Medicines administered through medicated gum and lozenges are absorbed through the buccal cavity, allowing for a fast onset of action. Lozenges are also available for a localised action, e.g. soothing and anaesthetising sore throats.

Currently, the only oral drug licensed in the UK that is administered within a gum formulation is nicotine. This chapter discusses the administration techniques used by nicotine gum.

It is advisable to inform the patient not to chew the gum continuously, as the nicotine is released too quickly and will then be swallowed. This can irritate the patient's throat, upset their stomach or give them hiccups. The 'chew and park' method is advised for this type of administration and is discussed in this chapter.[8]

Nicotine gum may not be a suitable administration method if a patient has false teeth. They may have difficulty chewing the gum, as it may stick to their false teeth.[8]

Lozenges may not be a suitable administration method if a patient is not able to hold a lozenge in their mouth and choking is a potential risk.

Oral powders/granules

Oral powders/granules are available as bulk (multi-dose) or unit-dose powders. Bulk powders are used less frequently. Often, a medicine spoon or a specially designed scoop (e.g. for Creon Micro) is utilised to measure the dose of powder or granules required. Precision of dosing can be more difficult when administering bulk powders, so usually these are used to administer drugs that are less potent, e.g. antacids.

Unit-dose powders and granules are pre-measured dosage forms. There are two types of unit-dose powders and granules: those that need to be added to water prior to administration and those that do not. Both administration methods are discussed in this chapter.

Unit-dose powders are convenient, as no measuring is required. They also allow flexibility with drug dosing, particularly for children.

Both unit-dose and bulk powders can be added to foodstuffs, but this should be in line with guidance from the manufacturer. This is useful, as the taste of certain oral powders/granules may be perceived to be unpalatable for some patients. This may affect patient acceptance and therefore adherence.

Powders have benefits as oral formulations. They are easier to store, more stable and less susceptible to degradation than oral liquids. This can also influence expiry dates, so they may have longer expiry dates than certain liquids.

Unit-dose powders are easily transportable. However, bulk powders are bulky (as expected) and may be inconvenient for patients to transport. When powders are orally administered, drug absorption is usually quicker compared to that of tablets or capsules.

Reconstitution of powders to form oral liquids

Pharmacists usually provide this type of medicine in its reconstituted form, and this is regarded as best practice. However, there may be legitimate reasons why patients or their carers may need to reconstitute powders prior to administration in exceptional circumstances. This chapter discusses how you would counsel a patient to reconstitute powders at home.

Powders requiring reconstitution often can settle in transit and over time. It is therefore good practice (unless the manufacturer's guidance suggests otherwise) to shake or tap the product before reconstituting. Once the product has been prepared and is in storage, the powder can settle at the bottom of the bottle. Therefore, it is good practice to shake the bottle (unless manufacturer's instructions specifically advise against) before administering the liquid.

Once reconstituted, the stability of the resulting liquid is different from the original powder. This might mean that the storage conditions for such products change, e.g. from a cool dry place to refrigerator storage. It also might change the expiry date of the product. The resulting liquid is usually less stable than the original powder formulation and therefore will often have a shorter expiry date – sometimes as short as seven days.

Oral tablet[1]

1. Ask the patient to make sure their mouth is moist with either their saliva or a drink of water.
2. Advise them to remove the tablet from its packaging.
3. The patient should place the tablet on the centre of their tongue. If the tablet is oval or caplet-shaped, then it should be placed in parallel with the length of the tongue, as this will aid swallowing.
4. Ask the patient to take an immediate sip of water to wash the tablet down their throat.
5. Step 4 can be repeated if the patient feels that the tablet has not been swallowed.
6. Advise the patient to take a drink of water to ensure that the tablet has been completely swallowed.

This guidance can be applied to capsules, caplets and other oral medicines formulated to be swallowed whole.

Oral liquid with a measuring spoon or cup

1. With the cap still in place, ask the patient to shake the bottle of liquid to ensure the contents are mixed or suspended (unless otherwise advised in the manufacturer's guidance).
2. Advise the patient to remove the cap from the bottle.
3. Inform the patient they should measure the recommended volume of liquid using a medicine spoon or a measuring cup.
4. Ask the patient to tip the contents of the spoon or measuring cup into the mouth and swallow the dose.

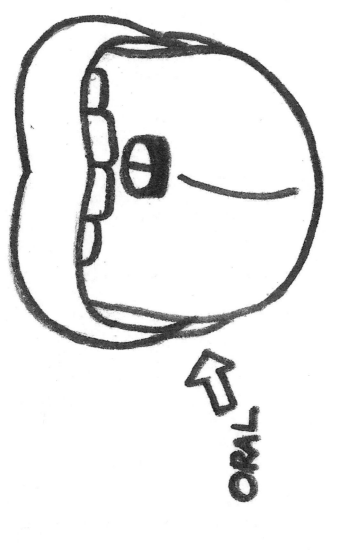

Figure 1.1 Administering an oral tablet.
Source: Jaspreet Bharaj.

5. Inform the patient they can take a drink of water to remove any lingering medicine taste.
6. Advise the patient to clean the neck of the bottle with a piece of damp kitchen paper, as this helps to ensure that the cap does not stick.
7. Ask the patient to replace the cap on the bottle and store as per the manufacturer's instructions.

Oral liquid with an oral syringe

1. With the cap still in place, ask the patient to shake the bottle of liquid to ensure the contents are mixed or suspended (unless otherwise advised in the manufacturer's guidance).
2. Advise the patient to remove the cap from the bottle.
3. Inform the patient they should insert the bung/bottle adapter (provided with the oral syringe) into the neck of the bottle. Ensure that this fits securely.[9]
4. Ask the patient to insert the oral syringe into the bung/bottle adapter.[9]
5. Advise the patient to invert the bottle so that the liquid moves to the bung/adapter end of the bottle.[9]
6. Inform the patient they should draw up the prescribed dose into the syringe by pulling on the plunger until the medicine reaches the required level. The top of the coloured ring (of the syringe) should be on the graduation mark of the dose required. Figure 1.2a shows the correct positioning.
7. Inform the patient that if there are air bubbles within the syringe, they can push the medicine back into the bottle and repeat step 6.

8. Ask the patient to turn the bottle back into its upright position.[9]

9. Advise the patient to remove the oral syringe from the bung/bottle adapter. In order to do this, it is best to hold the bottle with one hand and the syringe (not by the plunger) with the other hand.

10. Inform the patient they should put the tip of the syringe into the mouth and angle towards the sides (insides of the cheeks). See Figure 1.2b for correct positioning.

11. Ask the patient to push down gently on the plunger to administer the medicine to the insides of the cheeks. If administering large volumes or to younger children, the dose can be split and administered to each side of the mouth.

12. Inform the patient that the dose should not be administered directly to the back of the throat, as this will potentially initiate the gag reflex and cause choking.

13. Advise the patient to remove the syringe from the mouth.

14. Inform the patient that they can take a drink of water to remove any lingering medicine taste.

15. Ask the patient to remove the bung/adapter from the bottle.

16. Advise the patient to clean the neck of the bottle with a piece of damp kitchen paper, as this helps to ensure that the cap does not stick.

17. Ask the patient to replace the cap on the bottle and store as per the manufacturer's instructions.

18. Inform the patient that the bung/adapter and syringe should be washed after use as per the manufacturer's instructions.

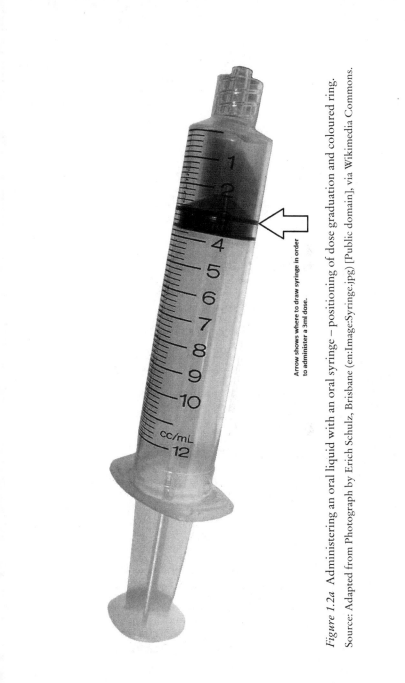

Arrow shows where to draw syringe in order
to administer a 3ml dose.

Figure 1.2a Administering an oral liquid with an oral syringe – positioning of dose graduation and coloured ring.

Source: Adapted from Photograph by Erich Schulz, Brisbane (en:Image:Syringe.jpg) [Public domain], via Wikimedia Commons.

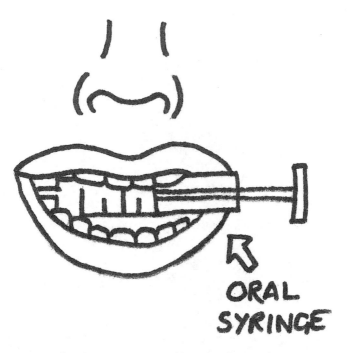

Figure 1.2b Administering an oral liquid with an oral syringe.
Source: Jaspreet Bharaj.

Buccal tablets

(Adaption based on review of patient information leaflets)[6,10,11]

1. Ask the patient to make sure their mouth is moist with either their saliva or a drink of water.
2. Using dry hands, advise the patient to place the buccal tablet between the gum and upper lip. The tablet needs to be positioned high up on the top gum. This can be placed on either side of the mouth. (See Figure 1.3.)

3. If the upper gum is not a comfortable position for the patient, e.g. due to wearing dentures, then the buccal tablet can be placed in any position between the gum and lip.

4. As the tablet begins to dissolve, it will soften and stick to the gum. Advise the patient not to chew or swallow the tablet, as it will need to completely dissolve and be absorbed through the buccal lining.

5. Advise the patient that they should not move the tablet with their tongue, as this will affect the rate at which it dissolves.

6. Inform the patient that it is advisable not to eat, drink, smoke or rinse their mouth whilst the tablet is dissolving and for a short period afterwards.

Buccal films have similar instructions to buccal tablets. However, the patient should be mindful of the positioning of film, e.g. a certain side may need to be placed against the mucosal surface.[12] Refer to specific patient information leaflets for this information.

Buccal liquid in pre-filled syringes

An example includes midazolam pre-filled syringes.

1. Advise the person administering to remove the oral syringe from its packaging.

2. Ask them to locate the buccal cavity – this is between the gum and the cheek. Do this by pinching and pulling back the cheek. An alternative method involves supporting the chin with one hand and pulling down

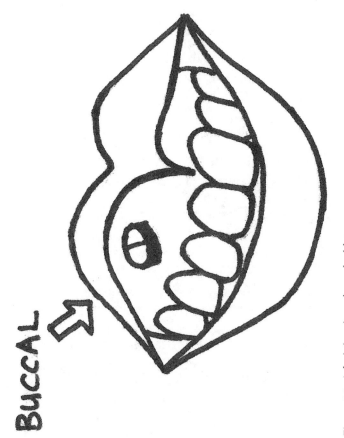

BUCCAL

Figure 1.3 Administering a buccal tablet.
Source: Jaspreet Bharaj.

gently on the lower lip. It is advisable to administer a liquid to the buccal cavity between the lower gum and the cheek. The syringe should not be put between the teeth.[7]

3. Advise the person administering to slowly push down on the pre-filled syringe plunger until the syringe is empty.[7]
4. If necessary, the dose can be administered in two parts, e.g. half a dose between each lower gum and cheek.[7]

Buccal liquid from multi-dose bottles using a syringe

An example includes midazolam multi-dose bottles (see Figure 1.4).

1. Advise the person administering to keep the bottle upright whilst removing the cap.
2. Whilst ensuring the bottle remains upright, ask the person administering to insert a syringe into its stopper.[7]
3. Advise them to carefully turn the bottle upside down.
4. Advise the person administering to pull down slowly on the syringe plunger and then push back, to release any air bubbles.
5. Ask them to slowly pull down on the syringe plunger until the required dose is measured.[7]
6. Inform the person administering to carefully turn the bottle back to its upright position and remove the oral syringe.[7]

7. Remind them to replace the cap on the bottle, to prevent the medicine becoming spilt.

8. Ask them to locate the buccal cavity – this is between the gum and the cheek. Do this by pinching and pulling back the cheek. An alternative method includes supporting the chin with a hand and pulling down gently on the lower lip. It is advisable to administer a liquid to the buccal cavity between the lower gum and the cheek. The syringe should not be put between the teeth.[7]

9. Advise the person administering to push down slowly on the syringe plunger until it is empty.[7]

10. If necessary, the dose can be administered in two parts, e.g. half a dose between each lower gum and cheek.[7]

Sublingual tablets

(Adaption based on review of patient information leaflets)[10,13,14]

1. Ask the patient to make sure their mouth is moist with either their saliva or a drink of water.

2. Advise them to remove the sublingual tablet from its packaging.

3. The patient should place the tablet under their tongue, as far back as possible (see Figure 1.5).

4. Inform the patient that they should allow the tablet to dissolve under their tongue. They should not move, chew or swallow the tablet whilst it is dissolving.

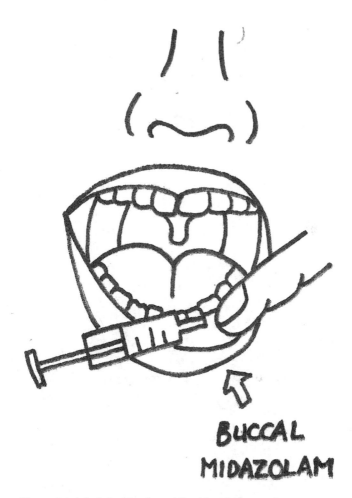

Figure 1.4 Administering buccal liquids using an oral syringe.
Source: Jaspreet Bharaj.

5. Inform the patient that it is advisable not to eat, drink, smoke or rinse their mouth whilst the tablet is dissolving and for a short period afterwards.

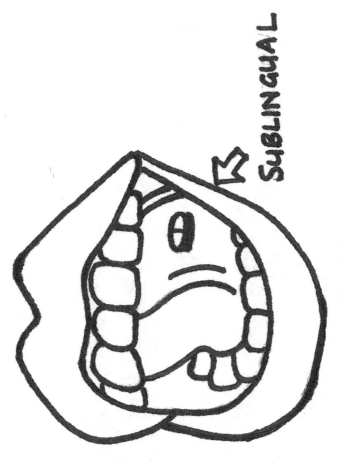

SUBLINGUAL

Figure 1.5 Administering a sublingual tablet.
Source: Jaspreet Bharaj.

Sublingual spray

(Adaption based on review of patient information leaflets)[10,15,16]

1. Before using the sublingual spray for the first time, advise the patient to prime the spray by spraying one dose into the air away from them.[14,15]
2. Ask the patient to open their mouth. Inform the patient that the spray should be held near to the mouth.[14,15]
3. Advise the patient to spray one dose under the tongue by pressing down firmly on the spray. The patient should avoid breathing in whilst spraying, so that they do not inhale the dose. This may be achieved by holding their breath immediately before spraying.[14,15]
4. Inform the patient they should close their mouth after spraying the dose.[14,15]
5. Ask the patient to repeat steps 2–4 if further doses are required.

Lozenge

(Adaption based on review of patient information leaflets)[10,17]

1. Ask the patient to place the lozenge into their mouth.
2. Advise the patient to put the lozenge between their cheek and gum, allowing this to dissolve slowly.

3. Inform the patient they should not bite, chew or swallow the lozenge whole.
4. Advise the patient to move the lozenge from time to time, from one side of their mouth to the other, until it is completely dissolved.

NRT lozenges

(Adaption based on review of patient information leaflets)[10,18]

1. Ask the patient to place the lozenge into their mouth.
2. Advise the patient to suck the lozenge until the taste becomes strong.
3. Inform the patient they should rest the lozenge between their gum and cheek.
4. Ask the patient to suck the lozenge again when the taste has faded.
5. Inform the patient they should repeat this routine until the lozenge dissolves completely (this should take approximately 30 minutes).

Medicated gum

(Adaption based on review of patient information leaflets)[8,10,19]

1. Ask the patient to place the medicated gum into their mouth.
2. Advise the patient to chew the medicated gum slowly until the taste becomes strong.

3. Ask the patient to 'park' the medicated gum between their gum and cheek.
4. Inform the patient they should chew the medicated gum again once the taste has faded.
5. Inform the patient they should repeat this routine until the medicated gum has lost its strength. This should take approximately 30 minutes.
6. When the medicated gum has lost its strength, advise the patient to remove it from their mouth and dispose of it carefully.

Reconstitution of powders to oral liquids

(Adaption based on review of patient information leaflets)[10,20]

As mentioned in the introduction, it is best practice to reconstitute powders to oral liquids when dispensing. However, there may be exceptional circumstances when a patient and/or parent, guardian or carer needs to do this at home.

1. Inform the patient the volume of potable water to be added to the powder.
2. With the cap still left on, ask the patient to tap the bottom of the bottle gently, to release any impacted powder.
3. Advise the patient to remove the cap from the bottle.
4. Ask the patient to measure the volume of water required using an appropriate measuring device,

e.g. oral syringe, measuring cup, conical measure. The powder should be left in its original container.

5. The solvent should be added to the solute – remind the patient to add the water to the powder, and not the other way around.

6. Inform the patient they should replace the cap and follow the manufacturer's instructions regarding the need to shake the product.

7. Advise the patient to follow the instructions for administering oral liquids (see earlier in this chapter) while following the prescriber's dosing instructions.

8. Inform the patient of any specific storage instructions and expiry dates as per the manufacturer's guidance.

References

1 NHS, Problems swallowing pills. Available from www.nhs.uk/conditions/swallowing-pills/Pages/swallowing-pills.aspx (accessed 14 December 2017).

2 Bandari S, Mittapalli RK, Gannu R. Orodispersible tablets: an overview. *Asian Journal of Pharmaceutics* (AJP). Free full text articles from *Asian J Pharm*. 2014 Aug 26;2(1).

3 Douglas L, Akil M. Sodium in soluble paracetamol may be linked to raised blood pressure. *BMJ*. 2006 May 11;332(7550):1133.

4 Siau K, Khanna A. Hypernatremia secondary to soluble paracetamol use in an elderly man: a case report. *Cases Journal*. 2009 Jun 29;2(1):6707.

5 Falagas ME, Vouloumanou EK, Plessa E, et al. Inaccuracies in dosing drugs with teaspoons and tablespoons. *International Journal of Clinical Practice*. 2010 Aug 64(9):1185–1189.

6 Teva B.V. Package leaflet: information for the user: Effentora® 100 micrograms buccal tablets, Effentora® 200 micrograms buccal tablets, Effentora® 400 micrograms buccal tablets,

Effentora® 600 micrograms buccal tablets, Effentora® 800 micrograms buccal tablets. Available at www.medicines.org.uk/emc/PIL.28855.latest.pdf (accessed 14 December 2017).

7   Great Ormond Street Children's Hospital, Buccal (oromucosal) midazolam. Available at www.gosh.nhs.uk/medical-information-0/medicines-information/buccal-oromucosal-midazolam (accessed 14 December 2017).

8   McNeil Products Ltd, Nicorette 4mg gum. Available at www.medicines.org.uk/emc/product/1323 (accessed 14 December 2017).

9   Great Ormond Street Children's Hospital, How to give your child liquid medicines. Available at www.gosh.nhs.uk/medical-information/medicines-information/how-give-your-child-liquid-medicines (accessed 14 December 2017).

10 Data Pharm, eMC. Available at www.medicines.org.uk/emc/ (accessed 15 December 2017).

11 Alliance Pharmaceuticals, Prochlorperazine 3 mg buccal tablets. Available at www.medicines.org.uk/emc/product/5227 (accessed 14 December 2017).

12 Meda Pharmaceuticals, Breakyl 200mcg buccal film. Available at www.medicines.org.uk/emc/product/5151 (accessed 14 December 2017).

13 Actavis Ltd, Buprenorphine 0.4mg sublingual tablets. Available at www.medicines.org.uk/emc/product/4271/pil (accessed 14 December 2017).

14 Indivior UK Limited, Temgesic 200 microgram sublingual tablets. Available at www.medicines.org.uk/emc/product/1142 (accessed 14 December 2017).

15 Aspire Pharma Ltd, Glyceryl trinitrate spray 400 micrograms/metered dose, sublingual spray. Available at www.medicines.org.uk/emc/product/674/pil (accessed 14 December 2017).

16 Aspire Pharma Ltd, Glytrin, 400 micrograms per metered dose, sublingual spray. Available at www.medicines.org.uk/emc/product/6692 (accessed 14 December 2017).

17 Teva Pharma B.V. Actiq 1200mcg lozenges. Available at www.medicines.org.uk/emc/product/6920/pil (accessed 14 December 2017).

18 The Boots Company Plc, Boots NicAssist 1 mg lozenge. Available at www.medicines.org.uk/emc/product/8344 (accessed 14 December 2017).

19 The Boots Company Plc, Boots NicAssist fruit fresh 2mg gum. Available at www.medicines.org.uk/emc/product/8349 (accessed 14 December 2017).

20 Kent Pharmaceuticals Ltd, Amoxicillin 125mg/5ml oral suspension BP. Available at www.medicines.org.uk/emc/product/2138 (accessed 14 December 2017).

2

Topical formulations

The topical preparations discussed in this chapter include creams, ointments, gels and lotions. Creams are multi-phase preparations, comprising of a lipid phase and an aqueous phase. Due to their aqueous content, patients often find these less greasy than ointments and therefore easier to apply. They have increased patient acceptability for daytime use, as they are less likely to stain clothing and they also feel lighter on the skin.[1]

Ointments are uniphase preparations within which solids or liquids are dispersed. Ointments are often firmer in consistency and greasier than creams, and thus tend to be less acceptable to patients for topical application. Some patients may prefer to reserve the use of ointments to night-time. They are particularly useful for dry skin, under wet wraps and when areas of skin have thickened, as they retain moisture well within the skin; this can promote repair of the skin barrier.[1] Some ointments contain paraffin. If the content of paraffin within a preparation is greater than 50%, then the ointment can be flammable. Patients should be advised to avoid smoking and naked flames. They should also be advised to change clothing and bedding regularly, as the paraffin can soak into these and make them flammable.[2]

Gels are liquids that have been formed into jelly-like formulations using appropriate gelling agents. They have a light and non-greasy feel that some patients find preferable to creams or ointments.[1]

Lotions are thinner than creams in consistency, as they contain more water than oil. They are easily applied and have a lightweight feel on the skin. They are particularly useful for hairy parts of the body.[1]

Other topical preparations available include pastes. These are not discussed in this chapter specifically; patients are recommended to refer to the specific manufacturer's guidance when administering these.

Topical preparations can be used to treat many local conditions, including: dry skin (e.g. as emollients), inflammatory conditions (e.g. steroid preparations), infections and allergies, etc. Some preparations may have multiple functions. For example, a cream may contain a steroid active ingredient in an emollient base. Some emollient products have antimicrobial and/or anti-itch properties – these are used to prevent infection and relieve irritation of dry skin conditions.

Patients using topical emollient formulations are recommended to use these frequently and generously to treat dry skin conditions – ideally every couple of hours, but at least twice a day. The frequency of administration may need to be increased in cold, windy or hot weather or when patients have a flare-up. Emollients cannot be overused.[1]

Patients should also reapply their emollient to damp skin after washing, showering and/or bathing. It is recommended that adults use at least 500g of emollient each week, whilst children should use at least 250g per week.[1]

When applying emollients, patients should be advised to apply in the direction of hair growth. This will minimise the risk of hair follicles becoming blocked and infected (folliculitis). Some patients may find it easier to apply topical emollients if they are warmed gently before use, e.g. by placing the container in an airing cupboard. Emollients should not be placed on a radiator or next to a direct heat source. When patients find that their skin condition is itchy and irritated, they may prefer to cool the emollient in the refrigerator (not the freezer).[1] Patients should check with the manufacturer's specific guidance regarding storage instructions, warming and/or cooling recommendations.

At night, emollients can easily transfer to bedding, particularly from the hands and feet. To prevent this, patients can be advised to wear cotton gloves and socks.

Some topical emollient preparations may also be used as soap substitutes. They do not have a foaming action; however, this is not necessary for cleansing the skin. They can be applied either before or during washing, showering or bathing, and then rinsed away. If patients are using emollients whilst washing, showering or bathing, they need to be aware that these may cause surfaces to become slippery. Extra care should be taken.[1]

Some topical products are susceptible to microbial contamination, and thus require preservatives to ensure an adequate shelf-life. Some patients might be sensitive to these preservatives. Preservative-free ointments are available and these may be useful to patients who experience sensitivities.

Whether or not the treatment is for infection, prudent hygiene measures should be followed when administering a topical formulation. These include washing hands before and after application. Soap substitutes can be used for this.

If patients have been prescribed large tubs of a topical formulation, it is advisable that they use a spoon to remove the quantity required and place it in a smaller clean container, e.g. a clean bowl. Any formulation remaining in the smaller container after application should be discarded. Patients should be advised not to use their fingers to remove the product from large tubs, as this can introduce microbes. Pump dispensers can minimise this risk of contamination. Patients should be advised never to share emollients.[1]

Patients using topical steroid formulations, e.g. creams and ointments, are advised to apply these sparingly, as they can cause thinning of the skin, 'stretch marks' due to a reduction in skin elasticity, and increased hair growth.[3] To advise patients on how much of their topical steroid to apply, a general guide has been devised, using fingertip units (FTUs). One FTU is the amount of cream or ointment that can be applied from the tip of an adult finger to its first crease – approximately 500mg of topical steroid.[4] Table 2.1 shows how much topical steroid (in FTUs) should be applied to each area of the body. The amount that should be applied to a child or baby is also described, using adult FTUs – however, the necessary quantity will be significantly less and will vary according to the child's age (see Table 2.2).[2,5]

Not all topical steroid formulations are equal in their potency – some are more potent than others. Figure 2.1 shows the different classifications of potency. Some drugs also have different strengths, e.g. Hydrocortisone 0.5% and 1%.

There will be many reasons why patients are prescribed topical steroids of different potencies. These include: age (children are usually prescribed weaker steroids); severity of condition; area and thickness of skin site needing to be treated (larger areas of skin may be treated with a weaker steroid, as may thinner areas of skin such as the face); and the need for bandaging (the occlusive nature of bandaging potentially increases the steroid potency, so a weaker steroid may be prescribed). Some patients may

Table 2.1 The number of fingertip units (FTUs) to be applied to an adult[2,5]

Area of body to be treated	Amount of topical steroid
Both sides of one hand	1 FTU
One foot	2 FTUs
One arm	3 FTUs
One leg	6 FTUs
Chest and abdomen (front of trunk)	7 FTUs
Back and buttocks (back of trunk)	7 FTUs

Table 2.2 The number of fingertip units (FTUs) to be applied to a child or baby[2,5]

Age	Amount of topical steroid				
	Face and neck	Arm and hand	Leg and foot	Chest and abdomen (front of trunk)	Back and buttocks (back of trunk)
3–6 months	1 FTU	1 FTU	1½ FTUs	1 FTU	1½ FTUs
1–2 years	1½ FTUs	1½ FTUs	2 FTUs	2 FTUs	3 FTUs
3–5 years	1½ FTUs	2 FTUs	3 FTUs	3 FTUs	3½ FTUs
6–10 years	2 FTUs	2½ FTUs	4½ FTUs	3½ FTUs	5 FTUs

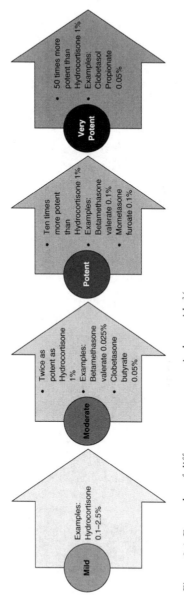

Figure 2.1 Examples of different-potency topical steroids.[3,6]

be prescribed multiple topical steroid formulations with different potencies, which may need to be used at different body sites.[3,6]

In order to prevent or minimise adverse effects, topical steroid formulations should only be applied to areas of skin affected by the condition. Adverse effects can also be minimised by using the appropriate quantity (in FTUs) of the lowest possible steroid potency and strength, for the shortest possible time. It is recommended by the British National Formulary that, as a general rule, topical steroid formulations should not be applied more than twice daily (often once daily is sufficient).[4]

Systemic absorption is a rare occurrence with topical steroid formulations. However, on rare occasions adrenal suppression and Cushing's syndrome have been associated with the absorption of potent and very potent topical steroids. Systemic absorption is highest in areas of the body where the skin is thin, or where the body rubs together (e.g. the skin folds of the breast or the digits of the hand). Absorption will also be greater where skin is damaged or irritated and under bandages or dressings.[6] Patients should be advised either to wear disposable gloves when applying topical steroids or to wash and dry their hands immediately after use.

When a topical steroid and emollient have been prescribed together, patients should be advised to leave a period of time between applying the two formulations. This is in order to prevent dilution of the steroid and it spreading to unaffected areas of the body. This period of time should be at least 15–20 minutes.[7] NICE Clinical Knowledge Summaries[8] and the Primary Care Dermatology Society[7] currently recommend applying the emollient first.

Cream, ointment or gel (from a tube)

(Adaption based on review of patient information leaflets)[3,6,9]

1. Inform the patient they will need to wash and dry their hands before administration.
2. Advise the patient to ensure that the area that they wish to apply the product to is clean and dry. This may mean that they need to wash the area(s). If this is necessary, advise the patient that they should not rub the area(s) dry. Instead, they should gently pat dry.
3. If this is the first time using the tube, advise the patient to check that the seal has not been broken.
4. Ask the patient to pierce the seal using the cap (turn the cap upside down and use the point to pierce the seal if necessary).
5. Inform the patient that they should apply the prescribed amount of product to the affected area(s) and gently rub into the skin in the direction of hair growth.
6. Ask the patient to wash and dry their hands (unless it is the hands that are being treated).
7. Advise the patient that they should replace the cap on the tube once application is complete.

Cream, ointment or gel (from a tub)

(Adaption based on review of patient information leaflets)[3,9]

1. Inform the patient they will need to wash and dry their hands before administration.
2. Advise the patient to ensure that the area that they wish to apply the product to is clean and dry. This may mean that they need to wash the area(s). If this is necessary, advise the patient that they should not rub the area(s) dry. Instead, they should gently pat dry.
3. If this is the first time using the tub, advise the patient to check that the seal has not been broken, if applicable.
4. Ask the patient to break the seal (if applicable), and remove the lid.
5. Advise the patient not to apply the product directly from the tub. Ask them to remove the prescribed amount using a spoon and add to a clean bowl.
6. Inform the patient they should apply the product to the affected area(s) and gently rub into the skin in the direction of hair growth.
7. Ask the patient to wash and dry their hands (unless it is the hands that are being treated).
8. Advise the patient they should replace the lid on the tub when finished and clean the spoon and bowl used.

Lotions

(Adaption based on review of patient information leaflets)[3,9]

1. Inform the patient they will need to wash and dry their hands before administration.
2. Advise the patient to ensure that the area(s) that they wish to apply the lotion to is clean and dry. This may mean that they need to wash the area(s). If this is necessary, advise the patient that they should not rub the area(s) dry. Instead, they should gently pat dry.
3. If this is the first time using the lotion, advise the patient to check that the seal has not been broken (if applicable).
4. If appropriate, ask the patient to break the seal or prime the pump following the manufacturer's instructions.
5. Inform the patient they should apply the prescribed amount of lotion to the affected area(s) and gently rub into the skin in the direction of hair growth.
6. Ask the patient to wash and dry their hands (unless it is the hands that are being treated).
7. Advise the patient that they should replace the lid/close pump when finished.

NB. Some lotions come with an applicator pad to apply the medication. Please follow the manufacturer's instructions for use.

Scalp application

(Adaption based on review of patient information leaflets)[6,9]

1. Inform the patient they will need to wash and dry their hands before administration.
2. Advise the patient to ensure that the area that they wish to apply the scalp application to is clean and dry. When the scalp application needs to be applied on hair-washing days, advise the patient they should ensure the hair is completely dry before administering.
3. If this is the first time using the bottle, advise the patient to check that the seal has not been broken (if applicable).
4. Ask the patient to break the seal (where necessary) and remove the cap following the manufacturer's instructions.
5. Advise the patient to turn the bottle upside down over the affected area(s) on their scalp.
6. Inform the patient to squeeze the bottle gently and dispense the prescribed amount onto the scalp.
7. Ask the patient to gently massage the scalp application into the affected area(s) to prevent 'run-off'. For some products this step is not necessary; refer to the manufacturer's instructions.
8. Advise the patient to allow the hair and scalp to dry naturally. Some products may feel cool on the skin until they have dried.
9. Inform the patient they should avoid touching their face and eyes until they have washed and dried their hands.
10. Advise the patient to replace the cap once finished.

Nail lacquer

(Adaption based on review of patient information leaflets)[9]

1. Inform the patient that they will need to prepare their nail before application. This is done by asking them to file the nail surface (including any infected or damaged parts). The file should not be used on healthy nails, as this may spread infection, and steps should be taken to prevent filing the skin around the nail.
2. Advise the patient to repeat step 1 for any other infected or damaged nails.
3. Ask the patient to clean the nail, using an alcohol swab or nail varnish remover on a cotton wool pad.
4. Inform the patient they should repeat step 3 for any other infected or damaged nails.
5. Advise the patient to open the bottle of nail lacquer.
6. Inform the patient to dip the provided applicator into the bottle. The excess lacquer should not be removed by wiping on the side of the bottle.
7. Advise the patient to apply the lacquer gently to the entire surface of the affected nail.
8. Inform the patient that the applicator is reusable; therefore, it needs to be cleaned using an alcohol swab.
9. If further nails require treatment, ask the patient to repeat steps 6–8 using a cleaned applicator each time.
10. Inform the patient they should allow the lacquer to dry completely before replacing their shoes and socks.

11. Advise the patient to replace the cap securely and to dispose of the alcohol swab/nail varnish remover pad carefully, as it is flammable.

For further applications to the same nail(s), the previously administered lacquer will need to be removed first using an alcohol swab or nail varnish remover on a cotton wool pad. The nail(s) should then be filed. Steps 5–11 can then be repeated.

Nail solution

(Adaption based on review of patient information leaflets)[9]

1. Advise the patient to open the bottle of nail solution.
2. Inform the patient to use the provided applicator to apply a thin layer of the solution to the affected nail and the surrounding skin. Repeat for other infected or damaged nails.
3. Ask the patient to wait 10–15 minutes before replacing their shoes and socks. Inform the patient that some nail solutions do not dry hard.
4. Advise the patient to avoid submerging their hands or feet into soapy water immediately after applying the solution. If the patient needs to wash up, then they should wear rubber gloves.

References

1 National Eczema Society, Emollients. Available at www.eczema. org/emollients (accessed 15 December 2017).

2   NHS, Fire hazard with paraffin-based skin products. Available at www.nrls.npsa.nhs.uk/resources/?entryid45=59876 (accessed 15 December 2017).

3   National Eczema Society, Topical steroids. Available at www.eczema.org/corticosteroids (accessed 15 December 2017).

4   British National Formulary, Hydrocortisone. Available at bnf.nice.org.uk/drug/hydrocortisone.htm (accessed 15 December 2017).

5   Henderson R. Fingertip units for topical steroids. Available at patient.info/health/fingertip-units-for-topical-steroids (accessed 15 December 2017).

6   British National Formulary, Topical corticosteroids. Available at bnf.nice.org.uk/treatment-summary/topical-corticosteroids.html (accessed 15 December 2017).

7   Primary Care Dermatology Society, Eczema – atopic eczema. Available at www.pcds.org.uk/clinical-guidance/atopic-eczema (accessed 15 December 2017).

8   NICE, Clinical Knowledge Summaries: eczema – atopic. Available at cks.nice.org.uk/eczema-atopic#!prescribinginfosub:6 (accessed 15 December 2017).

9   DataPharm, eMC. Available at www.medicines.org.uk/emc/ (accessed 15 December 2017).

3

Ocular formulations

The formulations administered to the eye and discussed within this chapter include: eye drops and ointments. Eye ointments are often oily, and are thicker in consistency than eye drops. They usually have a longer contact time with the eye, which means they do not need to be administered as frequently as eye drops. They are especially useful at night, as the long contact time means sleep is not disturbed by the need to administer the preparation multiple times. Ointments often cause blurred vision – therefore patients need to be cautious when driving or performing skilled tasks.

Eye drops often have a thinner consistency than eye ointments; however, viscous eye drops are available. Many patients prefer using eye drops to ointments, as they are less sticky and are less likely to cause blurred vision. Some drops can cause blurred vision and, if necessary, patients need to be advised on this.

Eye rinses and sprays are also available, for cleaning and lubricating the eyes. Patients should be advised to follow the individual manufacturer's instructions when administering such preparations.

It is important to check whether the intention is to apply eye ointments externally or internally. Some eye ointments should be applied externally, i.e. to the outer eyelid. For such cases, the ointment should be applied using a clean fingertip to the appropriate area of the eyelid(s).

Most ocular formulations exist as multi-dose preparations, but there are also unit-dose preparations available. These are often preservative-free and should be disposed of after administering the dose, as they are at increased risk of microbial contamination. Patients may be prescribed unit-dose preparations if they are allergic to preservatives.

Many multi-dose ocular preparations have a 28-day expiry date once opened. However, it is recommended to check the specific manufacturer's instructions for expiry dates and disposal information. It is good practice to advise patients to write the date of opening on the bottle, as this will help them to remember when to discard the product.

Ocular formulations may need to be stored at a range of different temperatures. Some preparations may require refrigeration (2°–8°C). The length of time in refrigerated storage may vary, e.g. some only require storage at 2°–8°C until they are opened for use. It is recommended to check the specific manufacturer's instructions for storage guidance.

Eye drops are available as solutions and suspensions. Suspensions will require shaking before use. This creates a uniform product, and thus ensures delivery of an accurate dose.

When multiple ocular preparations are being used by a patient, eye ointments should be administered once all eye drops have been instilled.[1] If multiple eye drop preparations are being administered, patients should be advised to wait 5 minutes between administering these.[2] This prevents the previous preparation being washed out by the next. If a long-acting eye drop needs to be administered with other eye drop preparations, this should be instilled last. This will make sure that the product does not get washed out by other preparations. Similarly, if a preparation causes irritation, this should be used last, to avoid tears washing out any consecutive drops.

It is recommended that patients do not use eye drops or ointments whilst wearing soft contact lenses. This is because some medicines and preservatives can build up in the lens, causing potential damage to the lens and eye. If soft contact lenses are required, they should be removed before the application of ocular preparations and then not reinserted for at least 15 minutes.[2,3] If patients use either hard or soft contact lenses, they are recommended to check with their contact lens provider and the medicine patient information leaflet for further information.

Whether or not the treatment is for infection, prudent hygiene measures should be followed when administering ocular formulations. These include washing hands before and after application. Prior to administrating eye drops or ointments, the patient should be advised to carefully clean their eye(s) if needed, as this will help to remove any discharge from the eye(s). Boiled and cooled water, or sterile sodium chloride 0.9%, or water for irrigation and a tissue or sterile gauze swab should be used to clean the eye. To avoid spreading infection, the patient should be advised to use a different tissue for each eye. Cotton wool is not recommended for cleaning eyes, as it may 'fleece' and irritate the eye.

To minimise the risk of the formulation draining down the back of the throat, the correct administration technique for eye drops is required. Poor technique is likely to result in the patient experiencing the taste of the drug as it passes down their throat.

Some patients may have difficulty self-administering eye drops. This may be due to manual dexterity issues such as poor grip strength or arthritis, or due to shaking hands, e.g. in neurological disease states. There are eye drop dispensers available that may help patients to retain their independence when instilling eye drops. Some patients may also find it difficult to ascertain whether or not an eye drop has been administered. By storing eye drops in the door of the refrigerator, the coolness of the drop may help patients to recognise that the formulation has already been administered to the eye.[4] Patients administering multiple ocular preparations, and who have difficulty distinguishing between them, may find it helpful to add different-coloured elastic bands to the bottles, which eases identification.

Ocular drops

(Adaption based on review of patient information leaflets)[5]

1. Inform the patient they will need to wash their hands prior to administration.
2. Advise the patient to sit or lie down, to aid successful administration.
3. Advise the patient to gently shake the bottle and remove the cap.
4. Ask the patient to tilt their head back and look up at the ceiling.
5. Advise the patient to pull down their lower eyelid gently to form a pocket between their eye and eyelid (see Figure 3.1).
6. Inform the patient to squeeze the upturned dropper bottle, to release a drop into the eye.
7. Advise that the patient places the drop into the gap between the eyelid and the eye.
8. The patient should avoid touching the dropper nozzle against their eye (or anything else).
9. Ask the patient to release the lower eyelid and close their eye (gently pressing against the corner of the closed eye where eye meets nose).
10. Advise the patient to wipe away any excess liquid from their cheek using a tissue or swab (they should not wipe near to the eye).
11. Ask the patient to press the eyelid gently at the inner corner of their eye for approximately 30 seconds, as this prevents the formulation draining to the tear duct and throat. This will help to reduce systemic absorption and a bad taste being left in the throat.
12. Ask the patient to repeat steps 4–11 for the other eye (if needed).

13. Inform the patient to replace and tighten the cap immediately after use.

14. Advise the patient that, if different ocular formulations are needed in the same eye, they need to wait 5 minutes before administering them.[2] This minimises the risk of the initial formulation being rinsed away, and thus not being absorbed.

15. If an eye ointment is required as well, the patient should be advised to administer this after all eye drops have been instilled.[1]

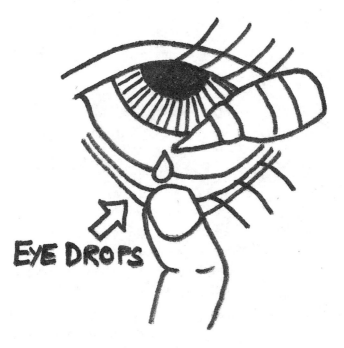

Figure 3.1 Administering ocular drops.
Source: Jaspreet Bharaj.

Ocular ointment

(Adaption based on review of patient information leaflets)[5]

If eye drops are also required, the patient should be advised to administer these before any eye ointments.

1. Inform the patient they will need to wash their hands prior to administration.
2. Advise the patient to sit down in front of a mirror.
3. Advise the patient to remove the cap of the tube.
4. If the ointment is to be applied inside the eye, advise the patient to pull down their lower eyelid gently, to produce a pocket space between the eye and eyelid.
5. Instruct the patient to squeeze the tube gently, to apply a thin ribbon of ointment (around 1cm long) into the gap between the eyelid and the eye. Start from the inner corner of the eye, next to the nose, and then move outwards.
6. Advise the patient to twist their wrist gently, to release the thin ribbon of ointment from the nozzle of the tube into the lower eyelid.
7. The patient should avoid touching the nozzle of the tube against their eye (or anything else).
8. Ask the patient to close their eye and blink, to spread the ointment over the surface of the eyeball. The patient may have blurry vision, but this will dissipate as the patient blinks multiple times.
9. Ask the patient to repeat steps 4–8 for the other eye (if needed).

10. Instruct the patient to replace and tighten the cap immediately after use.

11. Advise the patient that, if further ocular formulations are needed in the same eye, they need to wait 5 minutes before administering them.[1]

References

1 Moorfields Eye Hospital NHS Trust, How to use your eye ointment. Available at www.moorfields.nhs.uk/sites/default/files/how-to-use-your-eye-ointment.pdf (accessed 15 December 2017).

2 Moorfields Eye Hospital NHS Trust, How to use your eye drop. Available at www.moorfields.nhs.uk/sites/default/files/how-to-use-your-eye-drop.pdf (accessed 15 December 2017).

3 Rull G. Eye drugs – prescribing and administering. Available at www.google.com/url?q=https://patient.info/doctor/eye-drugs-prescribing-and-administering&sa=D&ust=1513342544105000&usg=AFQjCNFvwV8RvUSEcO30DMoNCegf_zEmPw (accessed 15 December 2017).

4 RNIB and IGA, Glaucoma focus. Available at www.glaucoma-association.com/glaucoma-focus/patient_literature.php (accessed 15 December 2017).

5 Data Pharm, eMC. Available at www.medicines.org.uk/emc/ (accessed 15 December 2017).

4

Aural formulations

Aural formulations are used to treat conditions locally within the ear. These conditions commonly include infections and an excess of earwax. Formulations administered to the ear and discussed within this chapter include drops and sprays. Ear washes – used for cleaning the ear – are also available. Patients should be advised to follow the individual manufacturer's instructions when administering such a preparation. Creams/ointments may be required to treat local skin conditions of the outer ear, and these will be applied topically.

Most aural formulations exist as multi-dose preparations. These often have a limited shelf-life once opened, e.g. 28 days. Patients are recommended to check the specific manufacturer's instructions, and also to refer to the manufacturer's guidance for specific storage recommendations for each aural formulation.

Ear drops and sprays are available as solutions, emulsions and suspensions. Emulsions and suspensions will require shaking prior to use in order to create a uniform product for delivery of an accurate dose.

Whether or not the treatment is for infection, prudent hygiene measures should be followed when administering an aural formulation. These include washing hands before and after application. Prior to commencing the administration of ear drops or sprays, the patient should be advised to clean their external ear carefully, if needed. This may be to remove any discharge from the ear(s), for example. The patient should be advised to use boiled and cooled water, sterile sodium chloride 0.9% or water for irrigation, and a tissue or sterile gauze swab to clean the external ear. To avoid spreading infection, they should use a different tissue for each ear as a precaution. Patients should be reminded to avoid inserting anything into the ear canal, e.g. cotton buds, as this can lead to damage to the eardrum. It is also important to follow the manufacturer's guidance on washing the device regularly, where necessary, to prevent microbial contamination.

Patients may find that the most comfortable position for administering ear drops is lying down on their side. They may find they need support from another individual to facilitate administration. To allow drops to soak in, the patient should be advised to stay on their side for 5 minutes.[1]

Some aural formulations contain arachis oil (peanut oil). The British National Formulary states that, as the oil is refined, it is unlikely to cause a reaction in patients with a known peanut allergy.[2] However, the Committee on Safety of Medicines (CSM) recommends that patients with a peanut allergy should not use medicines containing arachis oil.[3] In addition, some SPCs recommend that patients allergic to soya also avoid these products.

Swimming is not usually recommended whilst patients are being treated for ear conditions. If swimming is unavoidable, it is advisable to recommend that the patient wears a tightly fitted cap over their ears, to minimise water entering the ear. Patients should also try to avoid getting large amounts of water or shampoo or soap into the ear(s) when bathing or washing their hair, as this may further irritate the ear condition.[4]

Aural drops

(Adaption based on review of patient information leaflets)[5]

1. Inform the patient they will need to wash their hands prior to administration.
2. Advise the patient to shake the bottle gently and hold it in their hands for a few minutes to warm the formulation.
3. Ask the patient to remove the cap.
4. Advise the patient to lie down on the appropriate side (with the affected ear pointing to the ceiling) to aid successful administration. Alternatively, ask the patient to tilt their head to one side, with the affected ear pointing to the ceiling.
5. Advise the patient they should gently pull their earlobe backwards and upwards. This will allow the ear canal to be in the correct position for administering the formulation.
6. Instruct the patient to squeeze the upturned dropper bottle, releasing drop(s) into the ear.

7. Advise the patient to massage gently the front of the ear, adjacent to the ear opening.

8. The patient should be advised to remain lying down on their side or with their head tilted to one side for at least 5 minutes, to allow the ear drop(s) to enter the ear via the ear canal.[1]

9. Advise the patient to wipe any excess formulation away from the exterior of the ear, using a clean tissue.

10. Ask the patient to move into an upright position.

11. Ask the patient to repeat steps 4–10 for the other ear (if needed).

12. Ask the patient to wipe the dropper with a clean tissue after use and to replace and tighten cap (if present) immediately after use.

Aural spray

(Adaption based on review of patient information leaflets)[5]

1. Inform the patient they will need to wash their hands prior to administration.

2. Advise the patient to gently shake the bottle and hold it in their hands for a few minutes, to warm the formulation.

3. Ask the patient to remove the cap (if present).

4. Advise the patient to lie down on the appropriate side (with the affected ear pointing to the ceiling) to aid successful administration. Alternatively, ask the patient to tilt their head to one side, with the affected ear pointing to the ceiling.

5. Advise the patient that they should gently pull their earlobe backwards and upwards. This will allow the ear canal to be in the correct position for administering the formulation.

6. Instruct the patient to place the nozzle tip of the spray gently into the external ear, pointing towards the ear canal.

7. Advise the patient to press the nozzle once with their fingers, to release the spray. If further doses are required, advise the patient to press the nozzle again according to the manufacturer's instructions.

8. Advise the patient to massage gently the front of the ear, adjacent to the ear opening.

9. The patient should be advised to remain lying down on their side or with their head tilted to one side for at least 5 minutes, to allow the ear spray to enter the ear via the ear canal.[1]

10. Advise the patient to wipe any excess formulation away from the exterior of the ear, using a clean tissue.

11. Ask the patient to move into an upright position.

12. Ask the patient to repeat steps 4–11 for the other ear (if needed).

13. Ask the patient to wipe the nozzle with a clean tissue after use and replace cap immediately after use (if present).

References

1 Oxford University Hospitals NHS trust, Aural Care, West Wing: all about your ears – information for patients. Available at www.ouh.nhs.uk/patient-guide/leaflets/files%5C5280Pears. pdf (accessed 15 December 2017).

2   British National Formulary for Children, Frequently asked questions – clinical. Available at https://bnfc.nice.org.uk/about/frequently-asked-questionsclinical.html (accessed 15 December 2017).

3   Chapman V. Arachis oil in medicines – what are the risks of developing peanut allergy? UKMi Q&A 95.5 (UK Medical Information 95.5). Available at www.sps.nhs.uk/articles/arachis-oil-in-medicinesnwhat-are-the-risks-of-developing-peanut-allergy/ (accessed 15 December 2017).

4   NHS, Ear infections. Available at https://beta.nhs.uk/conditions/ear-infections/ (accessed 15 December 2017).

5   Data Pharm, eMC. Available at www.medicines.org.uk/emc/ (accessed 15 December 2017).

Nasal formulations

Nasal formulations are used to treat conditions both locally within the nose, e.g. nasal polyps, and systemically, e.g. migraine, nicotine replacement therapy and hormone therapy. The epithelial lining of the nasal cavity is thin, which allows for fast drug absorption. Nasal administration avoids hepatic first-pass metabolism, also reducing the time taken for a drug to act. This route may be particularly useful for drugs that are poorly absorbed or degraded by the gastrointestinal tract, e.g. hormone treatments.

Formulations administered to the nose and discussed within this chapter include nasal drops and sprays. Sinus rinses are also available – these are used for cleaning the nose. Patients should be advised to follow the individual manufacturer's instructions when administering such a preparation. Creams/ointments may be required to treat infections, and will be applied topically.

Most nasal formulation exist as multi-dose preparations. However, there are also unit-dose preparations available. Patients are recommended to check the specific manufacturer's instructions for the expiry date and disposal instructions, and also to refer to the manufacturer's guidance for specific storage recommendations for each nasal formulation.

Nasal drops and sprays are available as solutions and suspensions. Suspensions will require shaking prior to use in order to create a uniform product for delivery of an accurate dose.

Most multi-dose nasal sprays being used for the first time will need to be primed.[1,2,3,4] This can be done by spraying a dose into the air away from the face, as detailed within the individual manufacturer's instructions. In addition, if the nasal spray has not been used for a while, it should be primed again using the method described above.

Whether or not the treatment is for infection, prudent hygiene measures should be followed when administering a nasal formulation. These include washing hands before and after application. Prior to commencing the administration of nasal drops or sprays, the patient should be asked to blow their nose to clean their nasal cavity. If they are required to clean their nose, the patient should be advised to use boiled and cooled water, sterile sodium chloride 0.9% or water for irrigation. Patients should be reminded to avoid inserting anything into the nostrils, e.g. cotton buds, as this can lead to damage. It is also important to follow the manufacturer's guidance on washing the device regularly (where necessary), to prevent microbial contamination.

To minimise the risk of the formulation draining down the back of the throat, the correct administration technique for nasal sprays and drops is required. Poor technique is more likely to result in the patient experiencing the taste of the drug as it passes down the throat. If a patient experiences the taste of the drug, this can be alleviated by having a drink after administration.

Nasal drops can also be difficult to apply by oneself. Therefore, the patient may wish to ask someone to help them to administer this formulation.

When using nasal sprays, if more than one spray is required within the same nostril, it is recommended that the nozzle is angled in a different direction for the second spray.

Some nasal formulations contain arachis oil (peanut oil). The British National Formulary states that, as the oil is refined, it is unlikely to cause a reaction in patients with a known peanut allergy.[5] However, the Committee on Safety of Medicines (CSM) recommends that patients with a peanut allergy should not use medicines containing arachis oil.[6] In addition, some SPCs recommend that patients who are allergic to soya should also avoid these products.

Nasal sprays

(Adaption based on review of patient information leaflets)[7]

1. Inform the patient they will need to wash their hands prior to administration.
2. Advise the patient to gently shake the bottle and remove the cap.
3. Inform the patient they will need to prime the spray before use, as described in the introduction to this chapter.

4. Advise the patient to tilt their head slightly forward. They should do this by looking at their feet (see Figure 5.1).

5. Ask the patient to ensure that the bottle remains upright (see Figure 5.1).

6. Advise the patient to close one nostril, by applying gentle pressure against it with their finger. This should be the nostril that the spray is not being administered to.

7. Ask the patient to gently place the nozzle of the spray into their other nostril.

8. Inform the patient to breathe in normally through their open nostril and, at the same time, press the nozzle once with their fingers to release one spray. Advise the patient not to breathe in too hard, as they risk the dose being deposited at the back of the throat and this will reduce nasal absorption, and thus efficacy.

9. Ask the patient to remove the nozzle from their nostril and breathe out through their mouth.

10. The patient should be advised to tilt their head backwards, to reduce the risk of the spray running out of their nose and also to maximise absorption.

11. If further doses are required within the same nostril, advise the patient to repeat steps 4–10.

12. Ask the patient to repeat steps 4–11 for the other nostril (if needed).

13. After use, ask the patient to wipe the nozzle with a clean tissue and replace the cap immediately.

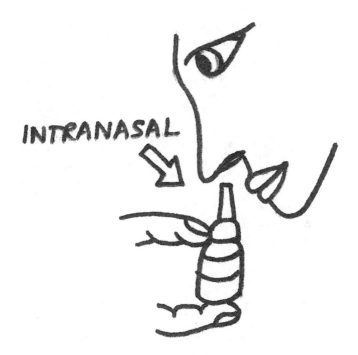

Figure 5.1 Administering a nasal spray.
Source: Jaspreet Bharaj.

Nasal drops

(Adaption based on review of patient information leaflets)[7]

1. Inform the patient they will need to wash their hands prior to administration.
2. Advise the patient to gently shake the bottle and remove the cap.

3. Advise the patient to lie down on their back with their head hanging over the bed. Alternatively, they can lean forwards, either by bending over or kneeling.
4. Advise that the patient places the required number of drops into the appropriate nostril.
5. The patient should avoid touching the dropper nozzle against their nose (or anything else).
6. Ask the patient to remain in position for a few minutes. This allows effective administration, and reduces the risk of the drops running down the nose or draining to the back of the throat. It should also aid absorption and reduce a bad taste in the throat.
7. Ask the patient to repeat steps 4–6 for the other nostril (if needed).
8. The patient should replace and tighten cap immediately after use.

References

1   GlaxoSmithKlein UK, Beconase aqueous nasal spray. Available at www.medicines.org.uk/emc/product/844/pil (accessed 15 December 2017).
2   The Boots Company plc, Boots hayfever relief 50 microgram nasal spray. Available at www.medicines.org.uk/emc/product/8305 (accessed 15 December 2017).
3   Aspire Pharma, Desmopressin spray 10 micrograms/dose nasal spray solution. Available at www.google.com/url?q=https://www.medicines.org.uk/emc/files/pil.8020.pdf&sa=D&ust=1513341401380000&usg=AFQjCNF45KFSaoLmsRyTiERHPV2WjrO7ug (accessed 15 December 2017)
4   Glaxo Wellcome SA, Pirinase allergy 0.05% nasal spray. Available at www.google.com/url?q=https://www.medicines.org.uk/emc/files/pil.4502.pdf&sa=D&ust=1513341401380000&usg=AFQjCNGxBxfMlUz4jd3LG28cqAETsvRpdA (accessed 15 December 2017).

5   British National Formulary for Children, Frequently asked questions – clinical. Available at https://bnfc.nice.org.uk/about/frequently-asked-questionsclinical.html (accessed 15 December 2017).

6   Chapman V. Arachis oil in medicines – what are the risks of developing peanut allergy? UKMi Q&A 95.5 (UK Medical Information 95.5). Available at www.sps.nhs.uk/articles/arachis-oil-in-medicinesnwhat-are-the-risks-of-developing-peanut-allergy/ (accessed 15 December 2017).

7   Data Pharm, eMC. Available at www.medicines.org.uk/emc/ (accessed 15 December 2017).

6

Inhaled formulations

Inhaled formulations are used to treat a number of respiratory conditions, e.g. asthma and chronic obstructive pulmonary disease (COPD). As the formulation is targeted to the area of treatment, smaller doses are often required and the risk of systemic side effects is minimised.

There are many different types of inhaler device. The most commonly prescribed inhaler is the pressurised metered dose inhaler (pMDI), also colloquially known as a 'puffer'. This device uses a propellant to release a suspension or solution of the drug into the lungs. pMDIs generally require coordination between the patient's inspiratory breath and the physical actuation of the device. Breath-actuated pMDIs are also available which remove the need for coordination. To be activated, these devices rely on the patient's own inspiratory breath.

Dry powder inhalers (DPIs) are also available. These use the patient's own inspiratory breath to propel a dry powder drug formulation to the lungs. There are many different types of DPI devices. In this chapter we discuss two of the most commonly used types: Accuhalers and Turbohalers.

If a pMDI is being used for the first time, it needs to be primed. The patient can do this by aiming the inhaler away from the face and pressing down with the finger(s) on top of the canister to release a puff of medicine. The number of puffs needed to prime the inhaler will vary depending on the device. The patient should be advised to check the specific manufacturer's instructions for their device. In addition, if the pMDI has not been used for a while, it should be primed again using the same method.

As the drug needs to reach the target site of the lungs, it is vital that patients have an appropriate technique when using their inhaler. Poor technique can lead to subtherapeutic doses, the swallowing of inhaled drug and can increase the risk of side effects, e.g. sore mouth.

Different devices will require a different inspiratory breath rate. Aerosol devices, such as pMDIs, require a slow and steady inspiration, whereas DPIs require a hard and fast inspiration technique. An incorrect inhalation rate may result in drug particles depositing at a non-targeted site. For example, inhaling pMDIs too quickly could result in an increase in the velocity of drug particles, leading to deposition on the throat. As DPIs do not have a propellant and require the patient's inspiratory breath to activate, inhaling too slowly may result in drug particles depositing within the mouth. A recent study found that 32–38% of patients using a DPI in the study had insufficient inspiration.[1] Devices, e.g. InCheck DIAL device and placebo inhalers, are available to help healthcare professionals coach patients in their inhaler technique and check their inspiratory rate.

Some of the most common technique errors include: poor coordination of physical actuation and inspiration of breath, resulting in the drug not reaching the target site; failure to prime the device before use, which may result in non-activation; failure to shake inhaler before use (if required), which may result in uneven dose distribution; and incorrect positioning of the inhaler, which may lead to escape of the drug before it reaches the target site. Other errors may include: failure to breathe out as fully as is comfortable before using inhaler, which may result in reduced space for the consecutive inspiratory breath; failure to hold breath after inspiration, which may result in reduced deposition of drug particles in the lungs; and omitting the wait period between actuations, which may result in reduced doses.[2]

As mentioned previously, poor technique can lead to an increased risk of side effects. This is a particular problem with steroid inhalers (for example, sore mouth caused by oral candidiasis). Patients should be advised to rinse their mouth, brush their teeth or gargle after using steroid inhalers. The use of spacer devices (as discussed below) can help with poor technique and also minimises side effects.

It is crucial that patients are provided with an inhaler device that is suited to their lifestyle, medical condition(s) and physical capacity, e.g. dexterity. This will ensure a greater level of patient acceptance and thus optimise adherence. Ideally, patients should be provided with placebo devices in order to trial their use, so they can make an informed decision regarding suitability. The UK Inhaler Group (UKIG) recommends that inhalers should only be prescribed when it is known that a patient can use the device.[3]

Patients should be advised on how their inhaler devices work and their frequency of use. For example, preventer devices, e.g. steroids such as beclometasone diproprionate, should be used regularly, as they reduce inflammation in the airways on a long-term basis, reducing bronchoconstriction. This can potentially decrease the need for acute relief. Relievers, e.g. short acting beta-agonists, such as salbutamol, reduce bronchoconstriction on a short-term basis and therefore are indicated for use in acute situations.

Patients should also be advised to keep spare reliever inhalers, where appropriate, so they have immediate access in an emergency. Patients should also be advised to be conscious of their inhalers' expiry dates (particularly if not used regularly) and the number of doses left in each device. This will prevent them from being without medication. Some inhaler devices have a dosing counter that indicates the number of doses remaining.

Inhaler devices require regular cleaning to ensure that dust or debris particles do not become deposited within the lungs. This will also help to prevent microbial growth, which could lead to local or systemic infections. Patients should be advised to follow manufacturer's guidance on how to clean their inhaler devices.

Spacers are empty, usually plastic, chambers that are used with pMDIs. There are two main types of spacer: large and small volume. They are also available with face masks for children and babies. Spacers are particularly useful for children, patients with high-dose corticosteroids, nocturnal asthma and patients for whom candidiasis with corticosteroids is an issue. The British National Formulary advises that larger volume spacers are more effective.[4] However, small volume spacers are also often prescribed due to their portability, which may improve patient acceptability.

As mentioned previously, spacers can help to improve technique and prevent side effects. Spacers hold drug particles within the chamber until the patient is able to breathe them in. This removes the need for coordination between the patient's inspiratory breath and the physical actuation of the device. Drug particles slow down whilst in the spacer, which means that patients do not need to worry about their inspiration rate. Patients may find that using a spacer leads to better control of their respiratory condition and a reduced need for multiple doses (this should be discussed first with their prescriber).

Spacers are generally easy to use. However, occasionally patients have issues when using them. The main issue associated with spacer technique occurs when patients fail to inhale their dose straight away after activating their inhaler. The drug particles will only stay suspended within the spacer chamber for a short period of time and, if there is a delay in breathing in, some of the dose may become deposited onto the surface of the spacer. This may result in sub-therapeutic dosing.

Failure to clean the spacer correctly can also lead to deposition of the drug particles onto the inner surface of the spacer chamber. Spacers should be cleaned monthly (this is contrary to some manufacturers' guidance) using mild washing-up liquid. Patients should be advised to allow the spacer to air-dry, as rubbing using a tea towel, cloth or kitchen paper, etc. can create an electrostatic charge.[5] This can pull the drug particles onto the surface of the spacer, which may result in sub-therapeutic dosing. The British National Formulary recommends that spacers should be replaced every 6–12 months.[4]

Pressurised metered dose inhalers (pMDI)

(Adaption based on review of patient information leaflets)[2,6]

1. Advise the patient they should take off the mouthpiece cover from the inhaler and check that the mouthpiece is free of objects.
2. If the inhaler is new, inform the patient they will need to ensure that it is primed, as detailed in the introduction to this chapter.
3. Ask the patient to shake the inhaler. They should do this a couple of times to ensure that the propellant and drug are well mixed and that any loose objects are removed.
4. Inform the patient they should breathe in and then breathe out as far as is comfortable. They should

place the inhaler mouthpiece in their mouth, between the teeth and above the tongue. The patient should close their lips firmly around the mouthpiece, but should not bite it.

5. Advise the patient to breathe in slowly and deeply and at the same time press down on the pMDI canister with their finger(s), to release one puff of medicine. They should continue to breathe in slowly and steadily.

6. Instruct the patient to remove the inhaler from their mouth and hold their breath for a few seconds (approximately 5–10 seconds) or as long as is comfortable. They should then breathe out slowly through their mouth.

7. If they require further puffs, ask the patient to wait for 30 seconds before repeating steps 3–6.

pMDI and small volume spacer

(Adaption based on review of patient information leaflets)[5,6]

1. Advise the patient they should take off the mouthpiece cover from the inhaler and check that the mouthpiece is free of objects.

2. If the inhaler is new, inform the patient they will need to ensure that it is primed, as detailed in the introduction to this chapter.

3. Ask the patient to ensure that the spacer is free from any objects.

4. Advise the patient to insert the inhaler mouthpiece into the end of the spacer. The opening of small

volume spacers is usually soft and rubbery to allow the mouthpiece to fit. The patient should ensure that the pMDI canister is in an upright position.

5. Ask the patient to shake the inhaler with the spacer attached. They should do this a couple of times to ensure that the propellant and drug are well mixed and that any loose objects are removed.

6. Inform the patient they should breathe in and then breathe out as far as is comfortable and then place the spacer mouthpiece in their mouth between the teeth and above the tongue. The patient should close their lips firmly around the mouthpiece, but should not bite it.

7. Advise the patient to press down on the pMDI canister with their finger(s), to release one puff of medicine.

8. Ask the patient to take one deep, slow breath. Some small volume spacers contain whistles that activate if the patient is breathing too quickly. An alternative method of inhalation is the tidal breathing method. Instead of one deep breath, ask the patient to take five normal breaths so that the drug enters the lungs.

9. Instruct the patient to remove the spacer from their mouth and hold their breath for a few seconds, or as long as is comfortable. They should then breathe out slowly. (This step is not necessary if using the tidal breathing method.)

10. If they need further puffs, advise the patient to wait for 30 seconds before repeating steps 5–9.

pMDI and small volume spacer with mask

(Adaption based on review of patient information leaflets)[5,6]

1. Advise the patient that they should take off the mouthpiece cover from the inhaler and check that the mouthpiece is free of objects

2. If the inhaler is new, inform the patient they will need to ensure that it is primed, as detailed in the introduction to this chapter.

3. Ask the patient to ensure that the spacer is free from any objects

4. Advise the patient to insert their inhaler mouthpiece into the end of the spacer. The opening of small volume spacers is usually soft and rubbery to allow the mouthpiece to fit. The patient should ensure that the pMDI canister is in an upright position.

5. Ask the patient to shake the inhaler with the spacer attached. They should do this a couple of times to ensure that the propellant and drug are well mixed and that any loose objects are removed.

6. Inform the patient that they should breathe in and then breathe out as far as is comfortable and then place the spacer mask over their face ensuring their nose and mouth are covered and there is a good seal.

7. Advise the patient to press down on the pMDI canister with their finger(s) to release one puff of medicine and to breathe in slowly.

8. Inform the patient that they should keep the mask held to their face for five to six breaths (tidal breathing

method). For best results, patients should be advised to breathe through their mouth. Some small volume spacers contain whistles that activate if the patient is breathing too quickly.

9. If they need further puffs, ask the patient to wait for 30 seconds before repeating steps 5–9.

pMDI and large volume spacer

(Adaption based on review of patient information leaflets)[2,5,6]

1. Advise the patient they should take off the mouthpiece cover from the inhaler and check that the mouthpiece is free of objects.
2. If the inhaler is new, inform the patient they will need to ensure that it is primed, as detailed in the introduction to this chapter.
3. Usually large volume spacers come in two halves that patients will need to put together. Ask the patient to ensure that the spacer is free from any objects.
4. Ask the patient to shake the inhaler. They should do this a couple of times to ensure that the propellant and drug are well mixed and that any loose objects are removed.
5. Advise the patient to insert the inhaler mouthpiece into the end of the spacer. The patient should ensure that the pMDI canister is in an upright position.
6. Inform the patient they should breathe in and then breathe out as far as is comfortable. They should

place the spacer mouthpiece in their mouth, between the teeth and above the tongue. The patient should close their lips firmly around the mouthpiece, but should not bite it.

7. Advise the patient to press down on the pMDI canister with their finger(s) to release one puff of medicine and to breathe in deeply through the spacer mouthpiece.

8. An alternative method of inhalation is the tidal breathing technique. Instead of one deep breath, ask the patient to take five normal breaths so that the drug enters the lungs.

9. Inform the patient to remove the spacer from their mouth and hold their breath for a few seconds (approximately 5–10 seconds), or as long as is comfortable.

10. The patient should be advised to breathe out slowly through their mouth. (This step is not necessary if using the tidal breathing technique).

11. If they require further puffs, advise the patient to wait for 30 seconds before repeating steps 4–10.

pMDI and large volume spacer with mask

(Adaption based on review of patient information leaflets)[5,6]

In this situation the patient will be a child, so advice will usually be provided to the patient's carer, e.g. their parent or guardian. However, it may be appropriate to advise some older children directly.

1. Advise the patient's carer they should take off the mouthpiece cover from the inhaler and check that the mouthpiece is free of objects.
2. If the inhaler is new, inform the carer that they will need to ensure that it is primed, as detailed in the introduction to this chapter.
3. Usually, large volume spacers come in two halves that carers will need to put together. Ask the carer to ensure that the spacer is free from any objects.
4. Ask the carer to shake the inhaler. They should do this a couple of times to ensure that the propellant and drug are well mixed and that any loose objects are removed.
5. Advise the carer to insert the inhaler mouthpiece into the end of the spacer. The carer should ensure that the pMDI canister is in an upright position.
6. Inform the carer that they should place the spacer mouthpiece mask over the mouth and nose, ensuring there is a good seal.
7. Ask the carer to encourage the patient to breathe in and out slowly and gently.
8. Advise the carer to press down on the pMDI canister with their finger(s) to release one puff of medicine.
9. Inform the carer to hold the mask and spacer in place whilst the patient breathes in and out normally for five breaths (tidal breathing method).
10. Advise the carer to remove the mask.
11. If the patient needs further puffs, advise the carer to wait 30 seconds before repeating steps 4–10.

Dry powder inhaler (Turbohaler)

(Adaption based on review of patient information leaflets)[6,7]

1. Advise the patient that they will need to remove the cap.
2. Ask the patient to hold the device upright and twist the base of the Turbohaler to the right, as far as it will go. They should then twist the base back towards the left until it clicks.
3. Inform the patient they should breathe in and then breathe out as far as is comfortable. They should place the inhaler mouthpiece in their mouth between their teeth and above their tongue. The patient should close their lips firmly around the mouthpiece, but should not bite it. Their fingers/ hand should not cover the air inlets when holding the device.
4. Advise the patient to breathe in quickly and deeply.
5. Inform the patient to remove the inhaler from their mouth and hold their breath for a few seconds (approximately 5–10 seconds) or as long as is comfortable. They should then breathe out slowly through their mouth.
6. If they require further doses, inform the patient they should wait for 30 seconds before repeating steps 2–5.
7. Advise the patient to clean the device, if necessary, and to replace the cap securely.

Dry powder inhaler (Accuhaler)

(Adaption based on review of patient information leaflets)[6,7]

1. Advise the patient they will need to open the Accuhaler using the thumb grip, pushing it away from themselves until it clicks.
2. Ask the patient to hold the device horizontally or upright and slide the lever down until it clicks.
3. Advise the patient that the inhaler needs to be in a horizontal position for inhalation.
4. Inform the patient they should breathe in and then breathe out as far as is comfortable. They should place the inhaler mouthpiece in their mouth between the teeth and above the tongue. The patient should close their lips firmly around the mouthpiece, but should not bite it.
5. Advise the patient to breathe in quickly and deeply.
6. Inform the patient to remove the inhaler from their mouth and hold their breath for a few seconds (approximately 5–10 seconds) or as long as is comfortable. They should then breathe out slowly through their mouth.
7. Ask the patient to close the Accuhaler using the thumb grip, as this resets the inhaler.
8. If they require further doses, advise the patient to wait for 30 seconds before repeating steps 1–7.

References

1 Price, DB, et al. Inhaler errors in the CRITIKAL study: type, frequency, and association with asthma outcomes. *Journal of*

Allergy and Clinical Immunology: In Practice. 2017 Jul–Aug 5(4):1071–1081.e9.

2 Murphy, A. How to help patients optimise their inhaler technique. *Pharmaceutical Journal.* 2016 Jul 297(7891).

3 Scullion, J, Fletcher, M, et al. UK Inhaler Group: inhaler standards and competency document (December 2016). Available at www.respiratoryfutures.org.uk/media/69774/ukig-inhaler-standards-january-2017.pdf (accessed 15 December 2017).

4 British National Formulary, Respiratory system, drug delivery. Available at https://bnf.nice.org.uk/treatment-summary/respiratory-system-drug-delivery.html (accessed 15 December 2017).

5 Asthma UK, Spacers. Available at www.google.com/url?q=https://www.asthma.org.uk/advice/inhalers-medicines-treatments/inhalers-and-spacers/spacers/&sa=D&ust=1513349102622000&usg=AFQjCNHOEC2o0jziQcXLAIsyuCCAQr2Fag (accessed 15 December 2017).

6 Data Pharm, eMC. Available at www.medicines.org.uk/emc/ (accessed 15 December 2017).

7 Asthma UK, Using your inhalers. Available at www.asthma.org.uk/advice/inhalers-medicines-treatments/using-inhalers/#Videos (accessed 15 December 2017).

7

Transdermal patches

Transdermal patches are used to manage a range of conditions, including pain, nausea, dementia and the menopause. Most patches are gradual release formulations, which contain the drug in either a matrix or reservoir within the patch.

Different patches have different rates of drug release. The most commonly available, are those that are changed every 24 hours/72 hours/4 days/7 days. It is important that patients are kept on the same type of patch in order to reduce confusion and in some cases to ensure continuity of the drug release pattern.

As patches are a slow release formulation, they take time to reach their steady state. Therefore patients should be advised that they may not experience an immediate effect. Patients prescribed patches for analgesia may require additional pain relief during this period.[1]

Prior to application of a patch, the skin should be washed with water. Soap or lotion should not be used to cleanse the skin. The patient should wait until their skin is cool after showering or bathing, before applying the patch. They should also avoid application of creams, oils, lotions, etc. after washing, as this will affect the adhesion of the patch to the skin.[1]

When opening the outer packaging, patients are advised to take care that the patch does not become damaged. It is recommended to avoid using scissors or knives to open the packaging. Patches should be applied whole, and not cut or torn in any way.[1,2] It is advisable to take care not to touch the sticky part of the patch when applying.

Patches should be applied to clean, dry, non-broken/scarred, hairless skin. If the area of application is hairy, then the excess hair may need to be removed before application, to optimise adhesion. Different patches have different recommendations on how to remove the hair – some recommend shaving, whilst others advise to clip or cut the excess hair. It is advisable to check with the product manufacturer's guidance if this is required.[1]

Different patches may have specific application sites. Some manufacturers may also specify sites to avoid, e.g. hormone replacement therapy (HRT) patches should not be applied on, or close to, the breast area. It is therefore advisable to check the manufacturer's patient information leaflet for specific product instructions. It is advisable to avoid applying a patch to an area of the body where friction is likely, e.g. the waistband of garments.[1]

The adhesive on patches does not generally cause significant irritation to the skin. However, if patches are placed at the same site each time, then this is more likely to occur. Irritation can be minimised by rotating the site of application. It is also important not to apply the patch to broken, inflamed or irritated skin, as this will also increase the chances of skin irritation.[1] Application to broken, inflamed or irritated skin can also affect the rate of absorption of the drug through the skin.

Heat can increase the rate of absorption of the drug via the skin. Whilst wearing a patch, it is therefore advisable that patients avoid hot-water bottles, saunas, steam rooms, hot tubs, spas and Jacuzzis, long hot baths, sunbeds, and excessive sun. There have been reported cases of death due to opioid overdose because heat increased the rate of absorption from opioid patches.[2]

Patches are generally waterproof enough to allow showering, bathing or swimming, but it is advisable to check individual patient information leaflets for specific information. When bathing or showering, do not scrub the patch.[1] As mentioned previously, it is not recommended to have long hot baths whilst wearing patches. It is also recommended that patients always check that the outer edges of the patch are sealed closely to the skin, to prevent water entering through air pockets.

If a patch is unintentionally removed from the skin, it is important not to use the same patch again. A new patch will need to be applied at a different application site. It is important to remove the patch on the original planned day.[1,2,3]

Transdermal patches

(Adaption based on review of patient information leaflets)[1,3]

1. Inform the patient that they will need to wash and dry their hands before administration.

2. Advise the patient to ensure that the area they wish to apply the patch to is clean and dry. This may mean that they need to wash the area.

3. Ask the patient to cut or tear open the protective sachet and remove the patch. Inform the patient that, whilst cutting or tearing, care should be taken not to damage the patch. Advise the patient to retain the sachet for destruction of the patch.

4. Inform the patient that the adhesive side of the patch is covered by a protective layer. Ask the patient to peel off one side of this protective layer, taking care not to touch the adhesive part of the patch.

5. Advise the patient that by holding the protective layer, they should stick the patch to the skin application site. They should then remove the rest of the protective layer, ensuring that the patch sticks to the skin.

6. Ask the patient to press down on the patch for 20–30 seconds to ensure the patch is stuck down flat without bumps or folds. Pay particular attention to the edges of the patch, to prevent it from being removed unintentionally.

7. Advise the patient to wash and dry their hands after applying the patch.

8. Inform the patient to make a note of the day that the patch was applied and to follow the prescribed instructions regarding how long to leave the patch in place.

Changing or removing transdermal patches

(Adaption based on review of patient information leaflets)[1,3]

1. Inform the patient that, when replacing the patch, they should remove the old patch first, in order to prevent overdose. They should not reuse the patch.
2. As the patch may still contain medication, advise the patient that they should fold the patch in on itself (adhesive side to adhesive side) and then place in the opened sachet.
3. Ask the patient to dispose of the patch in the household rubbish. If the patient is resident in a care home or healthcare setting such as a hospital or hospice, used and unused patches should be returned to a community pharmacy or disposed of in the appropriate pharmaceutical waste bin.
4. Inform the patient that some of the adhesive may remain on the skin after removing the patch. This can be removed with soap and water or baby oil. Nail polish remover or alcohol should not be used, as it can irritate the skin.
5. When applying the new patch, advise the patient to repeat the steps in the administering transdermal patches section, making sure to use an alternative skin application site.

References

1 Data Pharm, eMC. Available at www.medicines.org.uk/emc/search?q=patches (accessed 15 December 2017).

2 MHRA, Drug safety update: serious and fatal overdose of fentanyl patches. Available at www.gov.uk/drug-safety-update/serious-and-fatal-overdose-of-fentanyl-patches (accessed 15 December 2017).

3 All Wales Medicines Strategy Group, Safeguarding users of opioid patches by standardising patient/caregiver counselling (September 2016). Available at www.awmsg.org/docs/awmsg/medman/Safeguarding%20Users%20of%20Opioid%20Patches%20by%20Standardising%20Patient%20and%20Caregiver%20Counselling.pdf (accessed 15 December 2017).

8

Vaginal formulations

Vaginal preparations are used to manage or treat a range of different conditions, e.g. HRT and vaginal infections. They exhibit their action locally (within the vagina) and have limited systemic absorption. There are a number of different preparations available that can be used intra-vaginally; these include: pessaries, vaginal tablets, vaginal capsules and vaginal creams/gels. Creams are available as external and internal preparations. In this chapter we do not discuss the application of external creams.

Many of the different preparations used intra-vaginally are supplied with an applicator to aid administration. This may be pre-filled (single use) or reusable for multiple doses. It is recommended that pregnant patients should be cautious if using an applicator. Some women prefer to administer intra-vaginal preparations, such as pessaries, by hand when they are pregnant (see Figure 8.1).[1]

Whether or not the treatment is for infection, prudent hygiene measures should be followed when administering a vaginal formulation. These include washing hands before and after application. In addition to this, some women may feel more comfortable inserting their vaginal dosage form at night (subject to prescriber directions) and/or wearing a sanitary towel or liner in their

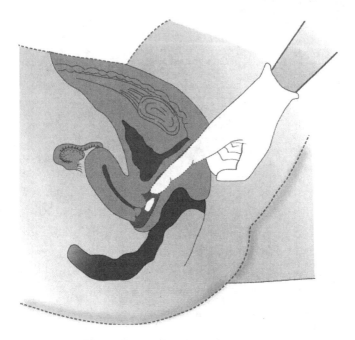

Figure 8.1 Administering medication vaginally without an applicator.

underwear for protection. This is because some vaginal products may leave a residue in the underwear. If a vaginal preparation needs to be used during a woman's menstruation, she should be advised to use sanitary towels, not tampons.

Patients also need to be advised that some vaginal preparations may affect the latex within condoms, caps and diaphragms, which potentially reduces their efficacy.

Alternative methods of contraception should be considered whilst using such vaginal formulations, and also for five days after their use. This advice does not apply to formulations designed for contraception.[2]

Polythene and PVC ring pessaries are also available to manage a uterovaginal prolapse. These are measured and fitted by healthcare professionals, and therefore the administration techniques discussed in this chapter are not applicable.

Vaginal pessary/vaginal tablet/vaginal capsule

(Adaption based on review of patient information leaflets)[2]

1. Inform the patient they will need to wash and dry their hands before administration.
2. Advise the patient to remove the applicator from the packaging and to pull the plunger out until it stops.
3. Ask the patient to remove the vaginal pessary/vaginal tablet/vaginal capsule from its packaging.
4. Inform the patient they should then insert the vaginal pessary/vaginal tablet/vaginal capsule into the holder end of the applicator. Some applicators will require the patient to squeeze the holder end in order to insert the vaginal pessary/vaginal tablet/vaginal capsule – check with the specific manufacturer's instructions.
5. It is important that the vaginal pessary/vaginal tablet/vaginal capsule is firmly situated inside the

applicator. However, advise the patient not to force it, in order to avoid the vaginal pessary/vaginal tablet/vaginal capsule becoming stuck within the applicator.

6. Advise the patient they should lie on their back with their knees bent upwards and spread apart.
7. Ask the patient to insert the applicator into the vagina as far as is comfortable.
8. Advise the patient to push the plunger until it stops to release the medication into the vagina.
9. Advise the patient to remove the applicator.
10. If the applicator needs to be used again to administer further doses, inform the patient to rinse it with warm water and dry thoroughly with kitchen paper before further uses.
11. If this is a single or final dose, the applicator needs to be disposed of in household waste.
12. Inform the patient they will need to wash and dry their hands after administration.

Vaginal cream/gel in pre-filled applicators

(Adaption based on review of patient information leaflets)[2]

1. Inform the patient they will need to wash and dry their hands before administration.
2. Advise the patient to remove the applicator from the packaging. With some applicators the patient will need to insert the plunger – check with the manufacturer's instructions.

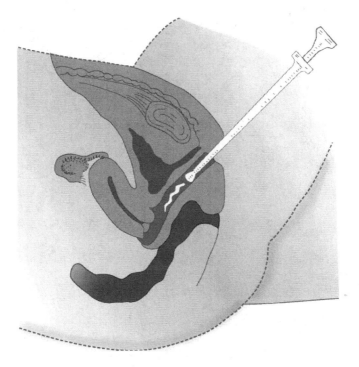

Figure 8.2 Administering medication vaginally using an applicator.

3. Ask the patient to remove the cap from the end of the applicator, taking care not to push the plunger in, so that cream/gel is not wasted.

4. Inform the patient they should lie on their back with their knees bent upwards and spread apart.

5. Ask the patient to insert the applicator into the vagina as far as is comfortable.

6. Advise the patient to push the plunger until it stops, in order to release the medication into the vagina (see Figure 8.2).

7. Advise the patient to remove the applicator.

8. Inform the patient that the applicator should only be used once and needs to be disposed of in household waste.

9. Advise the patient they will need to wash and dry their hands after administration.

References

1 NICE, Clinical Knowledge Summaries – candida – female genital. Available at https://cks.nice.org.uk/candida-female-genital #!scenario:4 (accessed 15 December 2017).

2 DataPharm, eMC. Available at www.medicines.org.uk/emc/search?q=vaginal (accessed 15 December 2017).

3 Rees Doyle G, McCutcheon JA. Administering medications rectally and vaginally. Available at https://opentextbc.ca/clinical skills/chapter/6-4-rectal-and-vaginal-medications/ (accessed 15 December 2017).

9

Rectal formulations

The rectum has a copious blood supply and avoids hepatic first-pass metabolism. It is a useful method of administration when the oral route is not appropriate, e.g. in patients who are nil by mouth or have dysphagia, and also in children. This means that often a smaller dose can be administered rectally compared with the oral equivalent. It is important to check the bioavailability of the drug when changing between these routes.[1] The rate of absorption can vary between rectal preparations.

Rectal formulations are used to treat conditions locally within the rectum and also systemically. Some of the local conditions that may be treated are haemorrhoids, constipation and inflammatory bowel disease. Systemic conditions that may be treated include status epilepticus, pyrexia and pain.

Rectal preparations include suppositories, enemas and rectal solutions. In this chapter we discuss the administration of suppositories. Enemas and rectal solutions have varying techniques depending on the product. Therefore it is recommended that the patient checks the specific manufacturer's guidance for information on administration.

Patients should be reminded that rectal formulations must not be swallowed and that all packaging should be removed carefully before insertion.

Prudent hygiene measures should be followed when administering a rectal formulation. These include washing hands before and after application. It is also recommended to advise patients to empty their bowels before administration, as an empty rectum will allow for better drug absorption. With the exception of laxative preparations, patients should try to avoid defecating for at least one hour after rectal administration.

Suppositories are designed to melt at body temperature (approximately 37°C). They should be warmed in the hand before insertion – however, not held for an extended period, as this may initiate the melting process. If patients find that the suppository is too soft for insertion before opening, they can place it in the refrigerator or under cold running water (whilst still in its immediate packaging).[2]

Patients may find that the most comfortable position for administering suppositories is lying down on their side. They may find they need support from another individual to facilitate administration, particularly in the case of children. An alternative method is to squat to allow administration. If a patient is having difficulty inserting a suppository, then a water-based lubricating gel may be used to aid administration.[3,4]

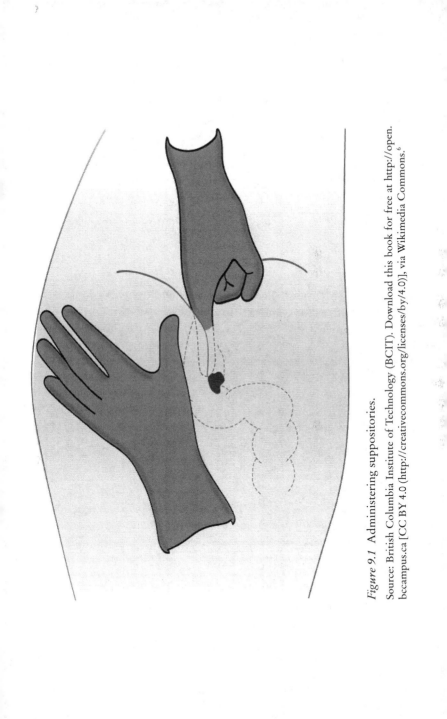

Figure 9.1 Administering suppositories.

Suppositories are 'bullet'-shaped with a rounded end and a blunt, squared end. It is usual to insert the suppository rounded end first (see Figure 9.1). However, if the suppository is expelled, then inserting it into the rectum blunt end first may help with retention. Placing the suppository against the wall of the rectum will also help the suppository to be retained for a longer period of time.[3,4] Patients should be advised to clench their buttocks together after insertion of the suppository into the rectum, as this also helps with retention.

As the suppository melts, some patients may find there is leakage from the anus. This can cause staining of clothing or bedding. Some patients may prefer to wear a pad in their underwear to prevent such staining and/or to insert the suppository at night (depending on the prescriber's instructions).

Suppositories

(Adaption based on review of patient information leaflets)[5]

1. Advise the patient to go the toilet and empty their bowels, if possible.
2. If necessary, ask the patient to clean and dry the anus area prior to administration.
3. Inform the patient that they will need to wash and dry their hands before administering the suppository.
4. Ask the patient to remove the suppository carefully from its packaging and warm it in their hands. It may

be necessary to apply a lubricant gel to the suppository at this stage, to aid rectal insertion.

5. Advise the patient to lie on their side and pull their knees towards their chest (if possible). An alternative position is the squat position.

6. Inform the patient to use their finger to insert the suppository gently into the rectum as far as is possible. This will aid with retention of the suppository in the rectum.

7. Ask the patient to keep the buttocks clenched together and remain lying on their side for several minutes (if the patient has chosen squat position, this does not apply).

8. Advise the patient that they should avoid emptying their bowels for at least one hour post-administration, if possible (if the suppository is for laxative use, this recommendation does not apply).

9. Advise the patient to wash and dry their hands following administration of the suppository.

References

1 Wright D. What is a suppository? Available at http://swallowing difficulties.com/healthcare-professionals/prescribing-different-formulations/what-is-a-suppository/ (accessed 15 December 2017).

2 American Society of Health-System Pharmacists, How to use rectal suppositories properly. Available at www.safemedication.com/safemed/MedicationTipsTools/HowtoAdminister/HowtoUseRectalSuppositoriesProperly (accessed 15 December 2017).

3 Norton C. The causes and nursing management of constipation. *British Journal of Nursing*. 1996 Nov 14;5(20):1252–1258.

4 Bradshaw A, Price L. Rectal suppository insertion: the reliability of the evidence as a basis for nursing practice. *Journal of Clinical Nursing*. 2007 Jan 1;16(1):98–103.

5 DataPharm, eMC. Available at www.medicines.org.uk/emc/search?q=Suppositories (accessed 15 December 2017).

6 Rees Doyle, G, McCutcheon, JA. Administering medications rectally and vaginally. Available at https://opentextbc.ca/clinical skills/chapter/6-4-rectal-and-vaginal-medications/ (accessed 15 December 2017).

Index